The Dating Dilemma

Handling Sexual Pressures

Bob Stone
and
Bob Palmer

Foreword by Jay Kesler

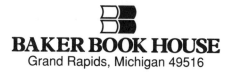

BAKER BOOK HOUSE
Grand Rapids, Michigan 49516

Illustrations by David Slonim

Copyright 1990 by
Baker Book House Company

ISBN: 0-8010-8314-1

Printed in the United States of America

Bob Palmer

has made major contributions to this book.
There is no question that he
deserves the title of coauthor.
However, to simplify and clarify the message,
both authors have chosen the "I" to be

Bob Stone

Contents

Foreword

The two Bobs—Palmer and Stone—are not theorists. A book like this could not be written by theorists. This book was birthed out of the combined almost forty years of day after day dealing with teenagers. The lives of Palmer and Stone back up their teaching. I trust them and have watched closely their personal growth and ministry. Few people in society are willing to lose their lives in the concerns and struggles of young people, but these two authors have. They have patiently listened to the trivial and the evasive and waited for the real problem to come up for discussion. They have sincerely prayed and studied their Bibles to help provide the answers that come not only from experience but also from the heart and mind of God.

The result is a truly moving and helpful book. Youth workers, pastors, teachers, counselors, and parents, as well as mature young people, will be helped by this book. All who read it will be well rewarded when they apply the lessons it contains.

Jay Kesler, President
Taylor University

1

The Biological
Hand Grenade Ladder

I do a lot of traveling. Recently, I boarded a flight and was seated beside a young couple who looked as though they might be on their honeymoon. The man had his hand on hers and was tracing small circles on her knuckles with his finger while they talked in hushed tones. Slowly, he moved his face closer and closer to hers. She seemed almost hypnotized by his comments and gestures of tenderness.

Suddenly the man reached up, took her face in his hands, and planted a long, lingering kiss on her lips.

Now I was sure they were newlyweds, probably on their way to a fancy hotel in Atlanta. I was somewhat surprised when I heard him ask, "What is your name?" His next question actually shocked me: "Are you stopping in Atlanta?"

She replied, "I could if you would like me to."

If, after this couple had spent a few hours together, we were to question them about their relationship with one another, they might tell us that they had fallen in love and that it was love at first sight. But is this actually possible?

The topic of this book is dating and sex, and our purpose is to help teenagers understand the importance of planting roots for right relationships. Exploring the many sides of love will be part of it.

An Embarrassing Topic

Most parents are painfully aware that the dating practices of a teenager largely determine the success or failure of an eventual marriage relationship. But parents are either too embarrassed to talk to their kids about dating and sex, or parents don't know how to clearly explain or define the dangers and difficulties of sexual involvement in dating. They wonder if their child will ask personal questions that they might be embarrassed or unable to answer.

I was speaking to a group of married couples at a retreat. One morning I announced that in the afternoon session I would be talking on "Sexual Harmony in Marriage." I suggested that those who might become easily embarrassed consider bringing a sack large enough to cover their heads so that others would not see their red faces. One man actually showed up for that meeting with a grocery sack over his head.

Why are we ashamed to talk about the beauty and importance of sex if God was not ashamed to create it? I don't think we should be.

The Ladder

In teaching teenagers about the patterns of sexual arousal and physical involvement, I use a diagram I call The Biological Hand Grenade Ladder. Before we look at the diagram I'll explain the terms.

Biology is the science of living organisms. Since a person is a living organism, and sexual response involves a person's body, it is logical to use the term *biological*.

A *hand grenade* is a very powerful explosive device. In the same way, sexual response, especially in a male, is powerfully explosive and often uncontrolled.

The concept of a ladder comes from the fact that sexual involvement is progressive. Each step leads to the next. This is the ladder of emotional and physical involvement. Here's how I diagram it.

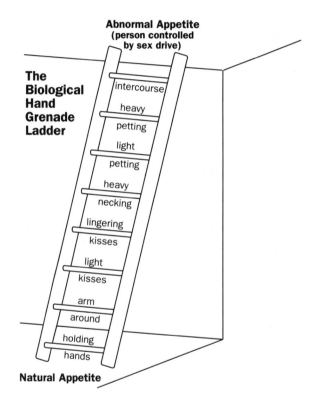

The appetite

At the bottom of the biological hand grenade ladder is the natural, God-given appetite. All of us are born with a certain natural hunger or desire for knowledge. Children are naturally curious. This is why they incessantly ask questions.

Your hunger for knowledge of and experience with sex is also a normal part of your growth. The Bible indicates that God's plan is that your sexual appetite should awaken gradually but be controlled until it is fulfilled and satisfied in a proper marriage relationship. But there is much to threaten and rush God's plan to a premature fulfillment. Because of the major emphasis on sex in our society, plus the push for younger and younger dating, children are taught how to arouse their natural passions to a level that quickly can be out of control. The entertainment media, too, gives visual and vocal enticement and explicit demonstrations on how to arouse passion in yourself and another person.

Holding hands

Teenagers like to hold hands. Young teens especially seem to hold hands a lot. This is the first step on the ladder of physical expression. Now, why in the world do kids enjoy holding hands so much? It feels good. There is a certain biological response inside each person when he or she first holds hands. Holding hands with someone to whom you are attracted creates a "warm, furry feeling" down inside.

In my studies of the human behavior of high school and college students, I have made this observation: If a guy is wise, he will watch a girl's facial response when he begins to attempt physical contact with her, or in other words, "when he puts the moves on her." If he reaches out to hold her hand, and she has a "glare like a groundhog," he is apt to stop and pull away; but if she responds with a pleasant look that communicates pleasure and approval, then he'll take her hand and squeeze it gently. From then on, wherever this couple is seen, they will probably be holding hands.

Some kids are embarrassed easily. One girl was embarrassed because her nervousness always made her hands sweat. She didn't think a guy would want to hold a girl's sweaty hand. She devised a remedy. She's the only girl I ever met who used antiperspirant on her hands.

Arm around

After a couple has been holding hands and enjoying the contact for a period of time, that special little thrill begins to wear off. The brand-new physical feeling seems to disappear, but something else is happening at the same time. They have a growing desire to show their affection for one another more aggressively. They want to be closer and more expressive. The guy has a built-in desire to put his arm around the girl, and the girl has an inner longing to be hugged by the guy she cares about. But because of the fear of rejection, they will usually proceed very cautiously.

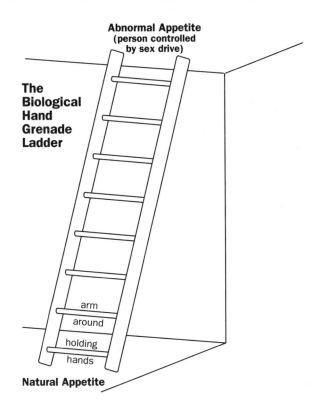

For instance, a guy will take a girl to a basketball game. As they sit on the bleachers watching the game (that is, he appears to be watching the game), the guy will be looking for an opportunity to "accidentally" put his arm around the girl's shoulder or waist. He sometimes uses what I call the "yawn-and-stretch method." He will stretch both arms above his head while yawning and then drop his arms, letting one fall around the girl. As he pretends to watch the basketball game, he actually watches her face to detect her nonverbal response when she feels his arm around her. If she grimaces or pulls away, he may say, "Oh, excuse me!" Or he may just remove his arm while his face changes color to "Alabama crimson." But if the girl smiles and appears to be enjoying the additional contact, the guy will probably keep his arm around her as long as he can.

The couple will be seen from then on in the school hallways or walking together along the street with the guy's arm around the girl's waist. Sometimes it is rather entertaining to watch two teenagers walking along with an arm around each other and holding hands. They can't walk normally and hang on to each other. It would almost require the agility of a contortionist to perform the physical activities some teenagers attempt to demonstrate their affection for one another.

What has happened? The couple has climbed to the second rung of the biological hand grenade ladder.

Kissing

The thrill of a guy placing his arm around a girl gradually begins to subside in him, while the desire for a more daring activity wells up. This moves the couple toward the third rung of the ladder—kissing. It is natural for a guy and a girl who are attracted to one another to want to be more and more expressive physically. Kissing is an intimate expression of affection. Again, because of the fear of rejection and failure, a guy will approach this phase of physical involvement with extreme caution, and so will a girl.

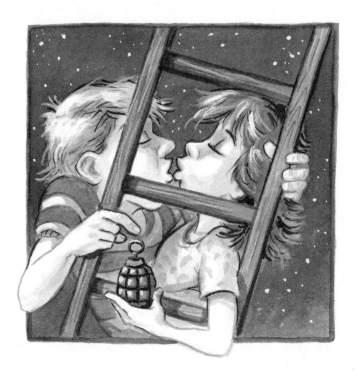

A guy wants to appear confident and experienced when he kisses his girl. He also wonders what it will feel like to press his lips to hers. So he begins to fantasize about kissing. Many guys will try to find a way to practice kissing before the actual event takes place. Several college men told me that as young teenagers they attempted to practice embracing and kissing, using such objects as pillows, mirrors, and even their own arms.

Terry practiced by kissing a mirror. He would try to see how he looked while kissing. He did this so often that it was practically a daily exercise. He said he felt like he was doing "lip push-ups."

The first time a guy kisses a girl, he is usually so shy that he will give her a quick peck, a "hit-and-run job." After a few of those quick kisses, if the girl does not resist his advances, a guy's confidence begins to grow. Once their natural desire for physical intimacy is aroused, the couple's kisses gradually last longer and longer.

Lingering kisses

The couple has now reached the fourth rung of the biological hand grenade ladder, lingering kisses. At last they have touched a tender nerve. They never before experienced such passionate pleasure. It was satisfying, in a way, to hug one another, but this . . . this is an indescribable experience! The sensations they feel in a lingering kiss are both pleasant and exciting. It feels so good they want to spend hours together just kissing. They seemingly forget eating and sleeping and homework and family responsibilities and everything else. They just want to sit in a romantic atmosphere and kiss.

But, this is the first major step toward an abnormal sexual appetite.

Am I saying that these desires and expressions are abnormal or unnatural? Not in the least. This is the natural sequence of progress in a romantic relationship. But now things get more serious.

Heavy necking

Lingering kisses trigger biological reactions that run deep within the body. Many young people say they experience chills down the spine and tingling sensations up the back of the neck and scalp. Some say they feel as if their hair is standing straight up on their heads!

With such physical responses so pleasurable, many people at this point disregard reason and simply give in to their natural desires. They ignore the guilt caused by extensive involvement. Beguiled by their emotions, teens are apt to rationalize that these physical activities are acceptable, because they think that they are in love.

Now on the fifth rung of the biological hand grenade ladder, the couple looks for opportunities to be alone. In a car, two teenagers can be isolated, anonymous, and incon-

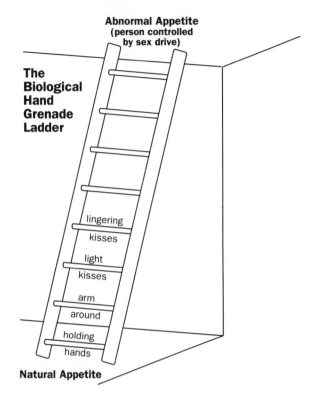

spicuous for hours at a time while they begin preliminary research in "oral communication."

After they reach this level of involvement, a couple is usually content to remain there for a while. They delight to experience a new degree of sexual awareness and experimentation. Other factors also may restrain further involvement: embarrassment, heavy guilt feelings, a fear of pregnancy (at least in the girl), or a compromised reputation, and fear of sexually transmitted disease.

Light petting

Eventually, a couple will discover that there are pleasurable sensations that result from touching and caressing. I tell teenaged girls that a guy's hands are "wired." A guy enjoys touching a girl's body.

A girl responds to touch. If a girl cares about a guy, she will be romantically aroused by his gentle caress. This is no surprise to God. In 1 Corinthians 7:1 the Bible says: "It is good for a man not to touch a woman." God gave this warning to the unmarried couple because he knew that touching would arouse sexual desires in both the man and the woman. Because God reserved sex for marriage, he cautions us not to arouse sexual desires in others that cannot be honorably gratified.

One guy asked, "How do you know it's okay in marriage, then?" The answer is in the very next verse. "Nevertheless, to avoid fornication [sexual immorality], let every man have his own wife, and let every woman have her own husband" (1 Cor. 7:2).

Now we've reached the rung on the biological hand grenade ladder called light petting. This activity, if continued, starts a couple down the road toward the major trap of physical intimacy. It may take days, weeks, or even months before they proceed, but eventually they will progress.

Now, you know you can't leave a plate of food in front of hungry persons and expect them not to eat it. If it sets in front of them long enough, they will catch a whiff of that delicious-smelling food. They will not be able to resist taking some.

In the same way, two teenagers cannot dangle the enticement of sexual pleasure before each other without eventually giving in to its allure. Proverbs 6:27 says: "Can a man take fire in his bosom, and his clothes not be burned?"

A guy will become bold and more demanding as he spends time alone with a girl. Her resistance will usually weaken with his persistence, because the desire for increased intimacy exists and grows in both of them.

Sherry, a fifteen-year-old, sobbed as she explained how she and Jeff had gotten so involved. "We spent a lot of time necking in his car on our dates. One night, after we had enjoyed an especially romantic evening together, he began to caress me. It felt so good I didn't want him to stop. When he touched my breast I was embarrassed, but it caused some very pleasant feelings. Even though I felt guilty, I let him continue. I told myself that it was not wrong, because we were so much in love with each other. After all, we were only expressing our love.

"I was surprised that when he touched my breast it caused feelings in other places. I wanted Jeff to go farther. Of course, I knew that I would never let him put his hand under my skirt, but I admit I wanted him to."

For several weeks after this, each of their necking sessions moved quickly to a petting session.

"One night after the basketball game, I was so proud of him because he had scored the winning points in the last ten seconds of the game. We were celebrating in every way we could think of. When we finally got alone and began to neck and pet, I got out of control. For some reason, I didn't care what he did, and I wanted to give myself to him in a special way. He suddenly touched my leg. I couldn't believe the pleasure I felt. I didn't even feel embarrassed. We went much farther than we should have, but I just could not bring myself to stop him.

"Later, when I was alone in my room, I had mixed emotions. I was embarrassed that I had gone so far. I was ashamed that I had disobeyed the Lord. I felt guilty for having enjoyed something that is supposed to be so sinful."

Sherry was totally unprepared for the allure of the pleasure that comes from physical involvement. She thought she could control her desires but discovered that they took control of her.

Heavy petting

When a couple reaches the rung on the biological hand grenade ladder labeled heavy petting, it is only a matter of time until they move on to the top rung of intercourse.

I was speaking to a group of nineteen hundred teenagers at a conference in Chicago. After one session, when all of the other young people were gone, one girl remained in the convention hall. Very shyly she approached me. With a stammering voice, hardly able to look me in the eye, she said, "I have one question I'd like to ask you."

In an effort to put her at ease, I jokingly said, "Well, I certainly hope it is not a very difficult question, because I'm not very smart."

After a nervous chuckle she asked, "Uh, well, uh, what is the difference between necking and petting?"

"Oh, that's an easy question. Necking is contact from the neck up, and petting is below the neck."

"Oh. Thank you very much," she called over her shoulder as she trotted away.

Neither kissing, necking, nor petting will afford a person any lasting contentment. A teenager may feel some degree of temporary enjoyment and gratification during these activities, but there will always remain a degree of unfulfilled desire, an unquenched thirst. There will be a craving to go farther to reach fulfillment and satisfaction.

Why do these enjoyable activities seem so incomplete? They were not meant to satisfy. God designed kissing and caressing, necking and petting to lead two marriage partners into the only sexual activity that does bring contentment—intercourse. But these activities were never designed to lead to that complete satisfaction outside of marriage.

"Outside of marriage," many teenagers will say. "Don't tell me you're a man who still believes that?"

Yes, I still believe that. After I made this statement to a high school class one day, a young man asked, "Am I understanding you to say that you do not believe in premarital sex?"

"You've got it, brother."

Immediately, about three-fourths of the class exploded into hysterical laughter, as if that were the funniest thing they had heard in a long time.

That experience reminded me that sometimes in life the right choice is not necessarily the popular choice.

I have been traveling all across America for a number of years trying to convince young people to wait until marriage to engage in sex. Many of them have laughed at me, thinking I'm out of touch with modern mentality. At the same time, billboards, TV soaps, commercials, magazine ads, rock groups, and even some of their peers have been telling them that premarital sex is not only acceptable, it is advisable. One of the most popular teen magazines in America has had articles encouraging premarital sex. An article in *SEVENTEEN* (August 1983, p. 86) clearly stated: "If the person and circumstances feel right, and if you are mature enough to take responsibility for your choice—not exploiting another person or taking unnecessary risks of pregnancy—you may be ready for sexual intimacy. But only you—not your peers—can judge whether that is true."

Now, however, due to the rapid spread of sexually transmitted diseases, many of these same sources are saying that the only "safe sex" is in a monogamous marriage with a partner who has also abstained before marriage.

Intercourse

The top rung on the biological hand grenade ladder is intercourse. When an unmarried couple climbs the ladder it leads to fornication: sexual intercourse between two unmarried people, which according to the Bible is sin.

In a proper marriage relationship, sexual intercourse can be one of the most deeply satisfying experiences a person can ever have. But outside of marriage it can be one of the most frustrating experiences. It can cause guilt, shame, fear, and resentment.

"Why did you marry Lisa?" I asked Todd.

"She sort of trapped me," he growled, resentment dripping from every word. "She led me into sex, and I felt obligated to marry her. Our sexual relationship seemed to be lacking something. I always felt guilty after sex. I thought that if we were married it would be more satisfying, because I wouldn't feel ashamed. Then, too, I was always afraid she might get pregnant."

Todd and Lisa had climbed the biological hand grenade ladder and were now reaping consequences in a miserable marriage where both of them were feeling cheated and unfulfilled.

The biological hand grenade ladder, then, is the physical and emotional process through which a couple moves from that innocent little activity of holding hands to the total physical commitment of sexual intercourse.

Where Sex Begins

Look again at the diagram of the biological hand grenade ladder. Where is sex on it?

Most teens will say, "Why, it's the top rung: intercourse." Ask parents the same question, and most will say that sex encompasses the entire diagram. Everything on the ladder is capable of causing or contributing to the arousal of sexual desire within a person. Obviously, that desire increases in intensity on each ascending rung of the ladder. When a guy and a girl are attracted to each other, any physical contact will be enjoyable and will create a desire for more. Each level never satisfies but leads to the next.

God's Design

Don't you think sex was a great idea? So do I. Sex was God's great idea, one of his gifts to humanity. His purpose for sex is both the continuation of the human race (called procreation) and the pleasure of a man and woman who are married to each other. Sex helps to deepen the marital relationship beyond any other relationship a person can have.

In creating and composing us, God designed our bodies

to respond in a progressive sequence to lead us naturally up the biological hand grenade ladder. It was God who created necking. He interrelated the sensual receptors, the nerve endings, with the emotions so that when two people press their lips to one another's there is a pleasurable feeling within them.

God created petting. Our creator designed us so that two people derive pleasure from touching one another's bodies. A woman especially responds to touch, and a man derives tremendous pleasure from touching a woman's body.

To engage in these activities in a dating relationship between two young people can be very frustrating, however, especially if at least one of them is determined to refrain from sexual intercourse until marriage.

It was probably this type of frustration that prompted the response of one young man in a psychology class where I spoke. I had just made the statement that God created necking and petting, when this high school senior blurted out, "You mean he gets the blame?"

"No, he gets the credit," I countered. "Whatever God does, he does well."

Planned Preparation

What, then, is the purpose for necking and petting? Is it intended to cause emotional frustration and physical suffering? Absolutely not.

God created necking and petting so that two married people can prepare one another's body for a very holy expression of their love for each other through the physical oneness of intercourse.

If God is the author of sex and its pleasures, and if he created it to be satisfying and fulfilling, why is it so confusing for dating relationships? Are there any guidelines for survival in this sea of discomfort and unrest? Absolutely.

2

Avoiding the
Wrong Perspective

You may be surprised, as I once was, to discover that the Bible has a lot to say about the subjects of love, sex, and marriage. There are three words in the New Testament that the Biological Hand Grenade Ladder is designed to illustrate.

Look again at the diagram of the biological hand grenade ladder.

Notice I have added three words that may be unfamiliar to you. Because these terms are not part of our everyday language, you might simply slide over them when you see them in the Bible.

Understanding words or phrases is basic to communication. Misunderstanding ranges from amusing to tragic. Beth had received a new snowsuit for her fourth birthday and was excited about getting to play in the snow. As the family drove into a shopping-center parking lot, Beth looked at the huge piles of snow scraped away from the building and heaped in ten-foot mounds along the edges of the lot.

"Oh, Mommy!" she exclaimed enthusiastically. "Can I slide down those big hills in my birthday suit?"

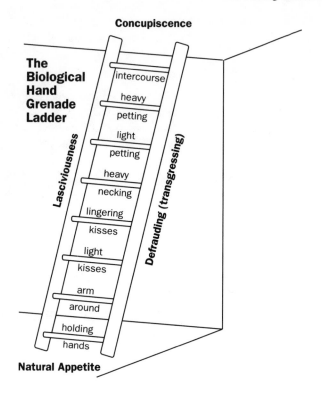

Wrong Desires

A clear understanding of terminology is crucial to comprehending a truth or a concept. It is essential for you to understand these biblical terms so you can grasp God's views on dating, courtship, and marriage. The words are *lasciviousness, concupiscence,* and *defrauding.* (These specific words are not used in all translations of the Bible but in those based on the King James Version.)

Lasciviousness

Notice that one of the legs of the biological hand grenade ladder is labeled lasciviousness. Lasciviousness is a likely result for a person who is involved in the activities listed on the rungs of the ladder.

What is lasciviousness? According to the dictionary, lascivious means "characterized by lust; lewd; exciting sexual desires."

Wait a minute! Is the dictionary saying that to stir up one's sexual desires is lewd or wicked? If so, then sexual desire is wrong and sinful. Is the Bible inferring that to have a desire for sexual fulfillment is evil? Not at all.

God says in Hebrews 13:4 (NKJV): "Marriage is honorable among all, and the bed undefiled; but fornicators and adulterers God will judge." Did you catch the contrast in that sentence? This verse gives us the key to the concept of lasciviousness. The Bible makes it clear that the marriage bed "is honorable among all." In other words, sex in a marriage relationship is right, honorable, and even holy, which is, remember, the theme of this book.

Illicit sex. The second half of the verse gives the warning against abuse of this principle: "but fornicators and adulterers God will judge." Fornication is sexual relations between a man and woman not married to each other. Adultery is defined as voluntary sexual intercourse between a married person and a partner other than the lawful spouse. In other words, a fornicator is interested only in self-gratification; an adulterer has broken his or her marriage vow to be faithful to the marriage partner.

By contrasting illicit sex with sex in its proper relationship, the Bible has defined the boundaries for sex as God intended it within marriage for the good of the partners, their families, and society.

The dictionary definition also uses the word *lust*. Lust is an overwhelming desire or craving, that is, a desire that becomes so powerful and consuming it begins to control the individual. It becomes a driving force, strong enough to compel a person to do things against his or her conscience.

Check out the word *lasciviousness* in Galatians 5:19 and you will see that it appears in a list of attitudes and activities that control non-Christians. These lifestyles are condemned by God. The Bible says that those who practice such things will not take part in God's kingdom. The word appears in a list of evil and immoral activities that have no place in the life of a child of God, for they can destroy a person both physically and spiritually.

Pornography encourages lasciviousness. "Bob, I can't help it. I'm oversexed." Tim sighed. "I just can't keep my hands off her."

Tim was a sophomore at the university. Shortly after he had committed his life to God, he started to date Ginger, who was also a Christian. They had recently become engaged. He came to see me because some of his attitudes and activities were causing problems on their dates. Ginger had explained to him that she was determined to refrain from sex until marriage. She said that, until recently, her love for him had been steadily increasing. Now, however, she was beginning to question the sincerity of his love for her. She did not want to do anything to jeopardize either their growing relationship or their future marriage.

Tim said that, because he loved Ginger, he wanted physical intimacy. In fact, every time they went out he tried to force her up the biological hand grenade ladder. She always resisted and kept saying, "Please wait." He kept pushing, because he thought she would eventually give in to his pressure. His persistence angered her. She finally became so upset with him that she told him if it didn't stop she would break their engagement and even quit dating him altogether.

As we talked about his problem of feeling "oversexed," he said that he had difficulty thinking about anything else.

"I can be sitting in class or even in church and be unable to concentrate on the lesson or the sermon, because I'm fantasizing about some sexual activity. It seems I can't look at a girl without wondering what it would be like to have sex with her," he confided.

"Do you read pornography?" I asked.

"Well, not as much as I did at one time," he admitted. "I

used to carry some 'girlie' magazines with me wherever I went. I don't do that anymore, but I still have some at home that I look at from time to time. Why, is that wrong?"

I explained that his reading pornographic material was stirring up his sexual appetite and leaving it unsatisfied and unfulfilled. He was also getting a distorted, selfish view of sex rather than developing the kind of understanding God wanted him to have about women and sex.

While pornographic literature is used by many guys to help them fantasize, girls will often begin with a romantic novel that may include graphic descriptions of sexual encounters.

The Bible says in Proverbs 23:7: "As [a man] thinketh in his heart, so is he." And Jesus said that if a man looks on a woman to lust after her, he has already committed adultery with her in his heart (see Matt 5:28). I believe the Bible is here teaching that "mental rehearsal" can be the same as "actual practice." For a great many, the "rehearsal" compels them to the "practice." When people fill their minds with descriptions of sexual activities, they will naturally look for the opportunity to have those experiences first-hand.

Furthermore, pornography encourages the selfish indulgence of men to exploit women and use them as playthings to satisfy their lustful pleasures. There is never any encouragement in pornography to build a deep, loving, permanent relationship based on mutual trust, commitment, and unselfishness.

Tim's attitude toward Ginger was one of selfishness. Yes, he cared about her, but he really wanted her to satisfy the sexual appetite that was controlling him. He had indulged in lasciviousness, and it was destroying his sensitivity to the needs and feelings of her and other girls.

When Tim realized that his lust was not only hurting Ginger and his relationship with her but also himself, he asked, "How can I be free from this bondage?"

I explained how to get down off the ladder, which we will cover in detail in chapter 9. He began to do the things I suggested, and finally he experienced the freedom to treat Ginger in a way that caused her love for him to grow deeper instead of growing cold.

So then, lasciviousness—selfishly stirring up sexual desire to satisfy one's own lustful appetites—is disturbingly related to the current attitude that "if it feels good, do it."

Concupiscence

Look again at the diagram of the biological hand grenade ladder. Notice that I have placed natural appetite at the foot of the ladder. The top of the ladder leads to concupiscence.

Concupiscence is a very strong or abnormal sex drive. It results from stimulating your sexual appetite over and over. Stimulating this appetite can be done through actual physical involvement with another person, or it can be done through fantasizing—mentally rehearsing sexual activities with someone. It is the point at which sex can be destructive.

The person who is controlled by concupiscence is not really interested in the other person but only in satisfying selfish lustful appetites. There is no sincere concern about the other person's future or feelings or family. This, of course, is the opposite of love. In his book *I Married You*, Walter Trobisch makes this statement: "Sex can be the death of love." You may wonder how this could be, for most teenagers equate sex with love. In a later chapter you will learn how sex can actually drive two people away from each other and even destroy love. But you can already sense this in the process of lasciviousness resulting in concupiscence.

At the same time these two things are taking place in you, something else is happening to the other person with whom you are physically involved.

Defrauding (or transgressing)

Check out the diagram of the biological hand grenade ladder again and you will notice that the other leg of the ladder is labeled defrauding (or transgressing), the third word from the Bible.

When you become physically intimate with someone of the opposite sex, ascending the biological hand grenade ladder and doing it on your own terms, you are not only stirring up and increasing your own sexual appetite, but you are also defrauding that other person. To defraud is to cheat or swindle. The guy, for example, is "cheating" the girl when he is stirring up appetites in her and implying that he is giving, or at least promising to give her, his love. Similarly the girl may defraud the guy. Sure, they may be able to satisfy their physical hunger for sex through intercourse, but there is an emotional and spiritual hunger that will remain unfulfilled apart from the commitment and working together in marriage.

Furthermore, extramarital intimacy is easily and casually dropped by one or both participants, and once that's done, easily taken up with another. But God wants sex to be a very special relationship between two marriage partners. If it is experienced with more than one person, it is no longer special. It loses some of its uniqueness, and then often, especially for a woman, sex can become a drudgery.

Some girls have been defrauded so much that they have lost their self-respect and their sense of right and wrong. They seem willing to do anything a guy wants them to do. They are either still seeking that elusive true love or no longer believing in it, and will go out and do these things with almost any guy. When the guys talk about dating a girl like this, they usually give her a nickname such as "Miss Warmth," because she seems to have no objections to anything they want to do. She is apt to end up the joke of the locker room.

Some girls do seem to have more inclination than others to "loose" moral standards. Since most girls by nature tend to be reserved about physical involvement, how does a girl become the type who will give herself freely to almost any guy she dates? There are several reasons this happens, but let's talk about two of the major ones.

Wrong Perspectives

Climbing the ladder

First, there is the climb up the ladder.

The ascent up the biological hand grenade ladder usually begins when a girl dates one guy on a steady basis for several months. As they get better acquainted, they become less inhibited and more involved. Perhaps their physical involvement will go as far as lingering kisses.

Mary Lou had long black streaks of mascara running past the corners of her mouth and falling as muddy droplets from her chin onto the table in my office. She had difficulty talking between her sobs.

"I . . . I'm . . . pregnant," she whimpered. "It will destroy my parents when they find out. I tried not to let it happen. Things just got out of control. What am I going to do?"

During the next weeks as we discussed her situation, Mary Lou retraced her steps and explained how she gradually moved into her present predicament.

"I dated Perry for over a year," she explained. "For a couple of months all he ever did was hold my hand or put his arm around me. Oh, he would give me a quick goodnight kiss, but that was all.

"Gradually, the kisses became longer. I thought we had a comfortable relationship. Then he met Barb and broke off with me. I was hurt but began dating Dan soon after our breakup.

"Dan kissed me the first time he took me out. By our third date we were into heavy necking. In a few weeks we began some light petting. At first, I felt terribly guilty and asked Dan to stop. But every time we went out, he would begin to pet, and each time I felt less guilty. Eventually, I ignored my guilt and felt petting was harmless. In fact, I thought it was only reasonable, because we were falling in love. We discussed it and decided petting was perfectly natural. We loved each other, so we shouldn't feel guilty. We thought somewhere along the way our parents had given us the old-fashioned idea that these things were wrong.

"I did draw the line at light petting, though. Dan got mad, but I refused to go farther. So he broke up with me. He said I didn't really love him or I would let him go farther.

"Then I met Pat. By our second date, we were petting. I was a little surprised, but it did seem sort of natural.

"I soon began moving the line on things I considered off limits because I really loved Pat and was convinced we would marry. Eventually, we wound up having sex every time we went out."

Mary Lou's experience is typical of many girls who are gradually led up the biological hand grenade ladder. When a girl responds to a guy's advances, in a sense she is "programming" her body. She is developing what psychologists call a conditioned response. For example, if a girl has previously been involved in petting, and a guy starts kissing her, she automatically anticipates and begins to have a desire for him to caress her. This then stirs up her desire for sexual fulfillment, for petting does not satisfy.

Obviously, the same type of responses develop in the guy who becomes physically involved with a girl. Once he has experienced the pleasures derived from petting, he is frantically dissatisfied with just kissing.

Craving affection

Jeff was a student at a small Christian college. He had a date with one of the secretaries who worked in the administration building. He was surprised when she got into his car and slid across the seat. She snuggled right up to him even before they left campus. He said, "I couldn't believe that woman. She acted as if she were starved for love." He later learned that she had grown up in a home without a loving father.

In contrast to developing a desire for sexual involvement through participation, a girl may feel a great need for physical affection because she came from a home where genuine affection was lacking. This is the second major reason a girl might give herself freely to nearly any guy she dates.

From my years in counseling, I've observed that if a girl is craving physical affection, it is very frequently because she did not have a good relationship with her father.

However, the opposite response can take place in some girls. When a girl grows up in a cold, indifferent home, she may have the same cold, unresponsive attitudes. One guy said that on a date, his arm accidentally touched the girl's elbow. She jerked away, looked at him with "a stare that could perforate my earlobes," and said icily, "Stop that! Watch it, Bud!"

He said, "For a minute there, I thought she was going to give me a karate chop."

There are three things, beside love and acceptance, that every girl needs from her father to develop a healthy, well-balanced response toward men: his attention, his affection, and especially communication.

Whether or not a girl comes from a home where she has a poor relationship with her father, if she dates a guy who begins to fulfill these basic longings or needs, she will want to respond to him. The guy communicates with her, and she loves it. He not only listens to her with interest and rapt attention, but he also shares some of his inner thoughts and feelings. I describe it this way: the guy "cracks open" his heart and lets the girl peek in to see what's inside. This openness and intimate sharing means a great deal to her, because it meets one of her basic needs.

A girl does not develop a need for communication only when she reaches her teens or when she becomes engaged. She is born with it. This is one reason guys think girls are nosy. It seems as if some girls have taken a course in police interrogation, because they are continually asking questions such as, Where did you go today? Whom did you see? What are you thinking about now?

A man sometimes feels like responding, "Woman, get away, will you? Where did you get all of these questions?"

I used to think that my wife was nosy until I realized that she asked so many questions because as a woman her desire to communicate expresses her need to nurture and show concern. Most men don't understand this basic need in a woman, because men do not have that need to the same degree. God created men with different needs, appetites, and desires from those he gave to women. Generally, young men especially are more interested in a physical relationship with a woman.

Wrong Behaviors

The experienced ladder climber

In addition to communicating with a girl, a guy will also show her some attention or thoughtfulness. He will send her cards or flowers, write her little notes, and call her on the telephone. He will stop whatever he is doing when she walks by so that he can "check her out."

The girl begins to feel worthwhile and important, possibly for the first time in her life. Now she is ready to respond to his efforts to show affection, particularly if she is starving for recognition. A girl will usually interpret all of these actions as love, but it may be that the guy is just using communication and thoughtfulness and showing her attention so that she will respond physically to his advances. In all of this, he is defrauding her.

There is a very thin line between sincere attention and fraud. The former is an expression of love and appreciation, but the latter is a deceitful means of exploitation. How do you tell the difference? One key test is self-restraint. If a guy sincerely cares about a girl, he will control his appetites and therefore his actions. He will show respect for the girl and refrain from intense physical involvement.

Of course, some girls also have an intense desire for a physical relationship. Consequently, they may encourage necking, petting, and intercourse. A girl will have greater respect and trust for a guy who will refrain from these activities, even though she desires and encourages it. She ultimately wants a husband in whom she can have complete trust and confidence.

Although a girl can defraud a guy, it tends to happen the other way around. This puts tremendous responsibility for thoughtful restraint on the guy—more difficult because it is less natural for him.

Dressing to defraud

How can a girl defraud a guy? A major way is by her style of dressing. She wears clothes that call attention to her body. Because men are visually oriented, they can be sexually stimulated by what they see. For example, when a guy sees a girl in skimpy or tight-fitting clothes, he will often be sexually aroused.

Teenage girls may think of such clothes as merely the height of fashion, but adolescent guys think those clothes are a sexual come-on. According to a survey of fourteen- to eighteen-year-olds conducted by four researchers at the

University of California—Los Angeles, boys still read more sexual come-ons into girls' behavior than the girls intend. They are likely to interpret a lowcut top, tight shorts or jeans, or no bra as deliberately enticing.

Girls do not fully understand a guy's response to visual stimulation, just as guys do not fully understand a girl's response to communication. Consequently, a girl may think that a guy is ridiculous in his response to the way she is dressed. Although most girls are conscious of attracting the attention of the guys by dressing "sexy," they may not realize that the attention they get will probably be from guys who want only their bodies.

To dress in an enticing way but have no intention of satisfying the desires that arouses in a man is dishonest. Teasing has its limits. Causing a guy to "fall in lust" with her and not "in love" is preying on his selfish desires and is a manifestation of her self-centeredness. Also, let this be a warning to the girl who naively dresses in an enticing way, for she unwittingly defrauds herself.

One girl could easily be responsible for defrauding dozens or even hundreds of guys simply by the way she dresses. All the guys have to do is see her.

But many girls would say, "Hundreds! I have not dated that many guys. I wish I had."

You don't have to date 'em to defraud 'em!

Defrauding spiritually

God has put into the heart of every girl a desire to have a spiritual relationship with the man she marries. She wants a man who will be totally open with her, who will share heart to heart. She wants a man who will put God at the center of his life and who will pray for her and with her. A woman usually has a more sensitive spirit than a man, and she will respond to a man who will be her spiritual partner and demonstrates spiritual sensitivity in their relationship. Because it is so unusual for a girl to find a guy who will take the lead in building their relationship with God at the center, a godly girl will be very responsive to this.

If a guy is sincere, this is beautiful. But some guys will take advantage of their response, and a girl needs to be alert to one who may be trying to deceive her.

Some guys are very skilled at deceiving a girl this way. In fact, the Bible says of certain ones: "Their eyes cannot look at a woman without lust, they captivate the unstable ones, and their techniques of getting what they want is, through long practice, highly developed" (2 Peter 2:14 PHILLIPS).

One girl was totally deceived by the "spiritual approach." She was on a date with a guy she thought was a fine Christian, and she had really enjoyed their time together. When they returned to her house, he suggested that they have prayer together before going in. She had never been asked to pray on a date and was nearly overwhelmed with excitement and gratitude.

The guy began to pray, and as he said, "Thank you, God, for Susie and for the wonderful time we have had together, etc.," he slowly put his arm around her and gradually drew her closer and closer.

Her heart began to pound, and her emotions raced. She thought she would melt right there in his arms. She felt an inner elation which she had never before experienced. When he kissed her, she had no desire to resist.

I believe that young man used prayer to defraud Susie. He deceived her into thinking he was building a spiritual base for their relationship, when actually he was maneuvering her into dropping her guard so he could lead her into physical involvement.

Prayer can melt the hearts of two people and unite them more quickly than anything else I know of. But Satan knows that, too.

More than one girl has told me how some guy misused Bible verses and twisted theology to try to convince her that premarital sex was morally acceptable.

Prayer is the most sacred and intimate link between God and people. Sex is the most sacred and intimate link in a husband-and-wife relationship. Satan is an imitator and deceiver, able to take any legitimate spiritual thing and design a conterfeit to corrupt God's great design and offer people an inferior substitute.

3

If It Could Happen to Him . . .

Just before midnight my phone rang. The voice on the other end was swollen with emotion. In near panic, the teenager pleaded, "What am I going to do? I just found out my girlfriend is pregnant. She refuses to have an abortion. I told her I would go with her to the abortion clinic and stay with her as much as they would let me. I promised her I would pay for it, too. But no matter what I say, she will not listen. I just can't reason with her. She is all emotional and cries all the time. She says the only solution is for us to run away and get married. She feels she just can't face her parents or her grandparents, especially her grandfather. Her grandfather thinks she is perfect. He is always doing special things for her. He told her recently he is going to buy her a real classy sports car when she graduates from high school. Now she won't graduate, unless she gets the abortion.

"If only I could talk her into an abortion!

"I can't run away and marry her. Things look real good for a four-year academic scholarship for me. Besides, my dad said that if I go to Purdue he will pay my way even if I don't get the scholarship.

"If only she would be reasonable and go for the abortion! She won't even go to one of those clinics to find out what is involved in an abortion. I told her that I heard about some drug a girl can take that will make her have a miscarriage, but she absolutely refuses to consider anything. She doesn't seem to understand that she is going to mess up both of our lives!

"She makes me feel so guilty. I've thought about suicide, but I couldn't do that to my mom and little brother.

"What can I do? I just can't stand the thought of not going to college and becoming an architect. That's all my dad has talked about since I was a little kid.

"I never dreamed things would get like this. I didn't think she would get pregnant. We tried to be careful."

A Dangerous Assumption

Teenagers assume that they are immune to this kind of situation. Most think it would never happen to them.

Many parents undoubtedly feel sure that such a thing would never confront their teenage sons or daughters. But if a young person chooses to climb the biological hand grenade ladder, there is a good chance that it will happen.

One of the effective deterrents to giving in to the allure of premarital sex is to learn about some of the devastating consequences of such activity.

One young man who was a very talented football player came to me for help. He had been dating one of the cheerleaders, who was also very popular in the school. He said that after they had been dating for several weeks, she invited him over to watch TV. Her parents had gone out for the evening, leaving the two teenagers alone in the house. She left the room where they were talking, and when she returned a few moments later, she was "indecently exposed."

"She was so gorgeous that I could not resist her advances," he lamented. "Now, I'm worried sick about the consequences."

David and Bathsheba

This young man's experience reminds me of an incident recorded in 2 Samuel 11.

She's beautiful

King David got out of bed one night and was walking around on the roof of his palace. It was probably the highest roof in the neighborhood. From his vantage point he could look down on all of the other homes. On this particular night he noticed a woman taking a bath on the roof of her house. He stood and watched her long enough to see that she was very beautiful. He decided that he would like to go to bed with her.

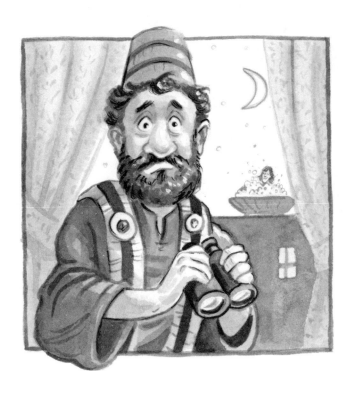

He asked his servants who she was. One of them told David that she was the wife of Uriah, a soldier in the king's army. David sent messengers to get her.

Now what do you suppose Bathsheba was thinking when the king's messengers showed up at her door at night, especially right at the time she was bathing?

Bathsheba probably said, "Why are you coming to my door at night while I'm taking a bath and I'm not dressed? Oh, the king wants to see me? At night?"

This situation raises some questions. For instance, why would Bathsheba be taking a bath on the roof of her house where she could be seen? Is it possible that she planned to be seen by King David? Did she know that he sometimes walked on the roof of the palace at night? Did she know exactly what she was doing, or was she completely naive?

Some girls seem to have what has been termed the "Hee-Haw Honey" syndrome. This concept comes from a television variety show featuring country music in a southern, rural setting in which a number of very attractive girls are dressed in such a way as to call attention to their physical attributes. Their attire is apparently intended to stir up lust in the men who see them, but the girls appear to be oblivious to the reactions of all the men around them.

Was Bathsheba infected with the "Hee-Haw Honey" syndrome? The Bible doesn't give us an answer.

Bathsheba must have been exceedingly beautiful for David to be willing to take the risks he did. He had at least eight wives, so it seems logical that he was not starving for sex. It was obviously not a matter of just satisfying his appetite with a woman; he wanted Bathsheba.

Bathsheba went to the palace, they had sexual relations, and she returned home. David assumed that this was the extent of his encounter with her. No one would ever know.

She's pregnant

A short time later, Bathsheba sent word to David that she was pregnant. Can you imagine the gut-wrenching panic he felt? What on earth could he do? She was married, but her husband was away in battle, fighting on behalf of the king. Uriah had not been home for several weeks and was not scheduled to return for several more.

David's servants knew that Bathsheba had been in the king's chambers late one night, and that her husband was away with the army. Unless David could devise a way to cover the natural consequences of his sin, the word would get out. Everyone would know that he had committed adultery with Bathsheba.

David probably did not sleep that night. Bathsheba was pregnant! He may have paced the roof of his palace trying to devise a way out. He may have stood in the same spot where he stood the night he saw her bathing, going over and over in his mind the events of that evening. He probably thought, It wasn't worth it. Why did I do such a foolish thing? Why did I risk my reputation for a few brief moments of pleasure? What can we do about her pregnancy? If only Bathsheba's husband would come home, even for a day or two. That's it!

Here's my plan

David had suddenly hit upon a plan to save his reputation and his "hide." He would call Uriah back from the battlefront for a report on the war "through the eyes of a foot soldier." David assumed that if he called Uriah home for two or three days, he would naturally go to his own house and have sex with his wife. Uriah would then go back to the battlefront. When he learned that his wife was pregnant, he would assume she had conceived the baby while he was home on leave.

Uriah did not conform to David's expectations.

When Uriah arrived, David asked about General Joab, the other soldiers, and the state of the battle. Then King David told Uriah to go home. David also sent a gift for Uriah to his house. But Uriah did not go home. He slept at the entrance to the palace with all of the king's servants.

The next day, when David learned that Uriah had not gone home, he summoned Uriah and asked him why. Uriah's response reveals such dedication and commitment that it should have pierced David's soul with shame and guilt. He explained that it did not seem honorable for him to sleep at home with his wife when the rest of the troops were sleeping in tents in an open field.

David was again panic stricken. He had not even considered that Uriah might not go home. The king now became desperate to get Uriah to sleep with Bathsheba. David invited him to dinner, where he got Uriah drunk. Surely Uriah would be too drunk to keep his commitment to the other soldiers.

Again David was wrong. Uriah slept with the servants.

The last resort

King David now began to lose control. He became reckless and violent with despair. He now would have to turn to his last resort: murder. David had allowed sin to gain complete control of his life. He was no longer in control of his heart and his life. He had become so shortsighted he was willing to "sacrifice the eternal on the altar of the immediate."

Can you believe this? He actually had Uriah, this faithful, honorable, dedicated soldier, whose commitment to the king was unquestionable, carry his own death warrant. David gave Uriah a letter to be taken to Joab, commander of the army. The letter instructed Joab to put Uriah in the most intense area of the battle. Then he was to withdraw the other soldiers so that Uriah would be killed. He was.

For the greater part of his life, David was one of the

most godly men recorded in Scripture. The Bible calls David a man after God's own heart. David knew God in a very personal, intimate way. He had a relationship with God that was unique. God spoke directly to him at times. David knew God's commands and the principles for overcoming temptation and avoiding sin.

Where the Battle Begins

How could a godly man like David be pulled so deeply into sin? David did not stop sin in its earliest stages. If he had handled the temptation in the right way, he would not have been shackled by lust, adultery, and murder.

At the very instant we are confronted with a temptation, we also sense an urging in our conscience to resist the temptation. In that split second, we make a decision about which impulse we will follow. We either give in to the temptation or we determine to resist it and do the right thing. If we determine to resist the temptation, there are some things we can do that will help us to maintain our commitment.

How should David have responded to his temptation? The very instant he saw that beautiful woman, he had a decision to make. He could continue to look at her and lust, or stop looking and walk away. He made the obvious choice to continue looking and to follow the path of lust. David knew the principle in Psalm 119:11: "Thy word have I hid in [my] heart, that I might not sin against thee." He also knew that a major way to resist temptation is to sing spiritual songs to yourself (see Eph. 5:18–19).

What a difference it would have made if David had said, "No, that is a trap. I will not walk into it." If he had begun to quote Scripture or sing his favorite song he could have redirected his thoughts toward the Lord. Then he would have had time and the presence of mind to consider the long-range consequences of giving in to lust.

If this sex-centered behavior could seize David's life,

don't you think it could happen to you? Many of us would be quick to respond, "It would never happen to me." But it is happening to people all around us who are just like us and who felt exactly the same way. You probably know someone who has fallen into sexual sin. You have probably seen some painful consequences in the life of that person and the lives of those who are close to him or her.

As a matter of fact, what you do in your dating relationships will affect your future marriage and your children.

"Aw, c'mon Bob," one guy chided, "everyone knows that sex is a private act between two people. You don't really expect me to believe that what I do in private with my girl is going to have any effect on the children I may have someday when I get married?"

Well, let's look carefully at some of the consequences of premarital physical involvement.

4

One Consequence
of Messing Around
Pregnancy

Using Birth-Control Devices

"We don't have to worry about pregnancy or sexually transmitted diseases because my girlfriend has an IUD," a college student said to me after I had spoken on dating and marriage in a class he attended.

What is an IUD? That is an intrauterine device, an object that is inserted in the cervix to prevent pregnancy. Many women have used them, but few know the facts about how they work or the risks in using them. At the outset, it should be clear that using an IUD will not prevent the transmission of a sexual disease.

James C. Upchurch, M.D., and I have offices in the same building. In an open letter he explains why he is opposed to the use of an IUD.

As you know, I practice obstetrics and gynecology in Birmingham, Alabama. When I became a Christian . . . the

51

Lord immediately began to deal with me in the area of abortions and intrauterine devices. I quickly realized that abortions under any circumstances amounted to murder, and the Holy Spirit also convicted me that the use of intrauterine devices for birth control was equally sinful.

In all types of IUDs studied, there is one common thread of similarity—they all seem to interfere with the implantation of the fertilized egg into the uterine cavity. It has never really been obscure to physicians that intrauterine devices abort rather than prevent pregnancy.

A pregnancy has existed for approximately six days when it reaches the cavity of the uterus. When an IUD is in place, the inner lining of the uterus is unable to accept the implantation of the fetus because of unfavorable chemical, hormonal, or inflammatory changes. Therefore, the intrauterine device could be more accurately classified as an aborting device rather than a contraceptive device.

It needs to be pointed out that there is a mortality rate associated with the intrauterine device, and there is also a hospitalization rate related to the complications of the use of the device. While IUDs are generally considered to be safe and effective by their proponents, there are significant complications which deserve to be considered: fainting (after insertion), perforation of the uterus, expulsion of the IUD, and a higher rate of pelvic infection.

After using an IUD, Dr. Upchurch says, "there is an increased problem of infertility." Physicians are aware that IUD use increases the risk of pelvic inflammatory disease (PID) with resulting scarring that may later cause difficulty in conceiving a child.

He also points out that there is a greater risk of tubal pregnancy, a pregnancy that takes place outside the womb. Finally, he says, "Many pregnancies associated with the IUD are complicated, and some have been associated with maternal death."

Rather than discussing the use of various other contraceptive devices such as the diaphragm, the now popular contraceptive sponge, the cervical cap, and the Pill, we would like to make three major points:

1. None of these devices is 100 percent effective. There is always a risk of pregnancy.
2. None of these devices protects against sexually transmitted disease.
3. These are methods used to bypass the results of activities in which a godly young person should not be involved. Protecting ourselves against the consequences of sin does not make our actions less sinful. God holds us responsible for our actions and for the attitudes of our heart.

Chances of Conception

"Aw, c'mon, man," one teenage guy moaned. "I'm not dumb. I'll be careful. Anyway, I heard that a girl can't get pregnant the first time she has sex."

In talking with the doctor mentioned earlier, I asked, "What are the chances of a girl getting pregnant the first time she has sex?"

He responded, "The chances are very high."

My wife, who is a registered nurse, also had thought the chances were low because of the emotionally tense atmosphere that usually exists in the circumstances surrounding the first time. However, the doctor believes there is at least an 80 percent chance for conception taking place. He added, "When a girl is ovulating, she is more affectionate and prone to respond romantically."

The other side of the situation to consider is that the average male ejaculates approximately 180 million sperm cells. Only one of those has to unite with the ovum for a girl to become pregnant. Those are pretty high odds.

One out of five teenage pregnancies happens within the first five months of the dating relationship. It doesn't take long to go up the biological hand grenade ladder, does it? I think the most logical conclusion to draw is not that it is an accident if a girl becomes pregnant during intercourse, but it is accidental if she does not get pregnant.

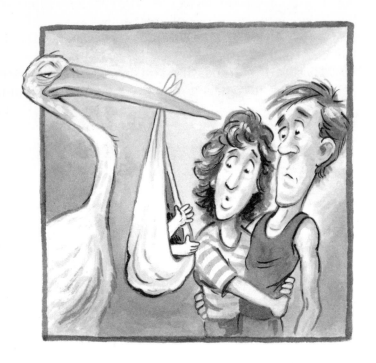

Pregnancy

Pregnancy is a major physical consequence of sexual involvement. To announce to the world that a woman is pregnant should be an exciting event. Unfortunately, many pregnancies are unplanned and/or unwanted. Recent (1990) statistics from the Alan Guttmacher Institute show that about 1 million teenagers have become pregnant every year since 1973. That's one out of ten girls ages fifteen to nineteen. A Department of Health and Human Service report (August 1990) indicated that one out of every four births in 1988 was to an unwed mother. The report goes on to say that there were 33.8 births per 1,000 population to teenagers ages fifteen to seventeen.

One day while talking with Dr. Upchurch I told him,

"Jim, I had the sad experience of counseling a fifteen-year-old who is unmarried and eight months pregnant." The doctor could identify with my feelings. At that time in his practice he had two pregnant fourteen-year-old patients and one who was only eleven years old. That little girl is too young to even begin to see the damage that has been done to her life!

What About the Baby?

Their age places teenage mothers at greater risk, and it is estimated that over 150,000 babies conceived by teenagers will die before or during childbirth. Teens also tend to be poor and are less likely to seek adequate prenatal care. Teens will choose to abort more than 400,000 of the babies they conceive.

The majority of the babies born to teenagers will have unwed mothers, and many will be given up for adoption. Of those who remain with their mothers, most will live in substandard or poverty-level conditions and will suffer serious health problems. They will not develop at a normal pace and will probably have social and academic difficulties in school. Often children of teenage parents drop out of school and become teenage parents themselves. One estimate states that 82 percent of girls who give birth at age fifteen or younger were themselves daughters of teenage mothers.

When Is a Baby a Baby?

The lady was crying when she walked up to me after I had spoken in her church. I asked why. She said, "Because my sister's fifteen-year-old daughter is scheduled for an abortion next Friday. I asked my sister why she would tell her daughter to abort her baby. My sister responded, 'Oh, it's not a baby yet.'"

Since teen sex frequently results in an unwanted pregnancy, what then? What do you face if it happens to you? Well, you are confronted with the same decision King David faced when he was unable to cover his sin with Bathsheba: whether or not to commit murder.

David had Bathsheba's husband killed. Today people have the unborn baby put to death. They don't call it murder. They don't even call the unborn child a baby; it is called a product of conception (POC).

The Bible says in Psalm 139:13–16 that God formed you in your mother's womb and that all of your attributes and characteristics were designed when you were still an unformed substance. You began when the sperm cell from your father met and united with the ovum (egg) cell from your mother.

As the nuclei of the ovum and sperm unite during the first hours of fertilization, they bring together twenty-three chromosomes from the mother and twenty-three chromosomes from the father. These chromosome sets carry some 15,000 genes from each parent cell.

In these first quiet hours of human conception, the genes, like letters of a divine alphabet, spell out the unique characteristics of the new individual. The color of the eyes and hair, skin, facial features, body type, and certain qualities of personality and intelligence are all determined by this genetic coding.

Do you want visible proof? Dig out your earliest baby pictures and the baby pictures of your parents or even your grandparents, and look at the striking resemblances.

One day a college student walked into Bob Palmer's office at the University of Arizona. Dropping a picture on Bob's desk, he said, "Look at this."

Bob commented, "That's a good picture of you, Brian. Where did you get those old-fashioned clothes?"

Brian said, smiling, "That's not me. This is a photo of my great-grandfather when he was about my age."

"I was astounded," Bob said. After he studied the photograph, it became obvious that it was not Brian, yet the resemblance was remarkable.

You see, your traits are determined not only by your parents but also by their parents and their parents before them. In fact, certain characteristics can be traced as far back as seven generations. I must believe that a baby is an intricately designed human being right from its conception. From the moment the egg is fertilized, the family characteristics from past generations are transferred to that microscopic embryo. The genetic code of the whole human being is contained in its first single cell.

Decisions, Decisions

When a dating couple learns that the girl is pregnant, they make a life-or-death decision concerning the baby —whether or not to have the baby aborted.

In the majority of cases, the girl wants to have her baby, and the guy insists on abortion. Often he is mainly concerned about being "found out" and having his plans altered. But for a girl there are more obvious long-term spiritual, psychological, and physical consequences to consider.

Counselors, social workers, and pastors say there are common reactions that almost always follow the same pattern in any girl or woman who experiences an abortion. Valerie's case is typical.

She was fifteen when she and Bill began to be sexually involved. At first she resisted Bill's attempts to caress her. But the longer they went together, the more difficult it became to resist his advances. Once she gave in, sex became a common activity on their dates.

When she gave up her virginity, she went home and cried most of the night. She had wanted to save herself for marriage. She determined that she would not allow things to go that far again. But with Bill's continual pressure and gentle persuasion, she began to give in quite often.

The day she was sure she was pregnant she told her friend Renee, who was three years older. Renee encouraged her to go to a clinic for crisis pregnancy counseling.

Abortion: The "Easy Way Out"

Bill took her to the clinic. The counselor at the clinic convinced her that an abortion was a simple solution to an otherwise major problem. Bill also insisted that an abortion was the only thing that could possibly make sense. After all, they were too young to get married, and it would upset both of their families if they found out she was pregnant.

Valerie was numb from all that was happening. She was confused, ashamed, and angry at Bill for pushing her into sex. She felt growing resentment toward him for being more concerned about his reputation than for the baby in her womb. She began to doubt his love, because he seemed largely unconcerned about her feelings.

The abortion was scheduled for two days later. Bill took her home and hurried back to school for basketball practice.

Valerie went directly to her room and cried uncontrollably, both out of fear and disappointment. She feared going through the abortion procedure, but she was also afraid of the reaction of her parents if they discovered that she was pregnant. She knew her mother would be heartbroken, but she thought, *Dad will get so mad that I don't know what he might do. He might go over and beat the thunder out of Bill.*

Her deep disappointment was due to Bill's lack of real concern for her feelings and the physical dangers she faced. She had been told by the counselor at the abortion clinic that this was a relatively safe procedure but that there are a small percentage of girls who experience resulting physical problems.

The risks

Valerie was given a single sheet of paper that outlined possible complications, including death, resulting from an abortion. The technical language was hard to understand. Besides, it scared her to think about what could go wrong. She folded the paper and put it in one of her books so that it would not be found.

Valerie should have given more attention to the possible complications of abortion. If she had, she probably would have decided not to go through with it. Psychologist Wayne R. Krug has written a pamphlet, *Abortion: Your Risks* (Birmingham, AL: Birmingham 1000 for Life). One of the statements he makes is: "Three out of four women who have abortions (77 percent) experience acute grief reaction." This is the intense kind of grief that people encounter whenever a loved one dies and, in the case of abortion, it is often accompanied by profound guilt for having abandoned her baby. (The mother who has an abortion may not necessarily feel that she has killed her baby. She may blame the abortionist for this.) Krug goes on to say:

> One out of two women who will have an abortion will experience emotional and psychological disturbances lasting for months which may include depression, insomnia, nervousness, guilt, and regret.
>
> Complications in future pregnancies will happen to one in four (24.3 percent) women which include such things as excessive bleeding, premature delivery, cervical damage, and sterility.
>
> One in six (17.5 percent) will have a miscarriage during her next pregnancy.
>
> There are additional side effects such as: 140 percent greater risk of breast cancer following an abortion, 30 percent increased risk of tubal pregnancy after one abortion, and 160 percent after two or more. Placenta previa, a condition producing extremely severe, life-threatening bleeding has an increased risk of 600 percent following an abortion.

Several groups of women are at significantly higher risk for postabortion problems. These women should be particularly aware of the greater potential for complications. Women under twenty have two times greater risk for medical complications than women aged twenty-five to twenty-nine. They also have 150 percent greater risk of cervical injury than women over thirty years of age.

One thirteen-year-old girl in Alabama had an abortion. She went directly to her bedroom when she came home. She began hemorrhaging but was afraid to tell her parents about the abortion. She died in her own bed, alone even though her parents were in another part of the house.

Getting back to Valerie, she slept very little the next two nights. Several times she decided to phone Bill and call off the abortion, but each time she would think of the problems her pregnancy would create for her family. She then convinced herself that she had to go through with it.

The clinic

The waiting room in the clinic was typical of any medical clinic, with one notable exception: All of the patients were teenage girls.

Bill was the only boy there. Valerie felt a slight sense of relief in that she wasn't all alone like the rest of the girls. She was encouraged a little by the fact that at least he cared enough to stay with her. The nurse had given her a shot when she arrived, which made her feel woozy and a little less apprehensive. When Valerie got on the table in the procedure room, she felt almost as if this were happening to someone else.

Valerie tried to push away the thoughts of an actual baby growing inside her. She kept thinking of it as only a "small blob of tissue," a concept she had received from the counselor at the clinic.

When the doctor came in, he was cool and very "clinical." He turned on a vacuum machine that was so loud it reminded her of the big vacuum her dad used to clean up sawdust in his basement workshop. When the doctor inserted the tube of the vacuum into her womb, she would hear the "whomp, whomp" of something being sucked through the tube. She felt her heart pound as she began to worry about what was actually happening to her. She wondered if this powerful machine could cause damage to her reproductive organs so that she might not be able to have a child someday when she and Bill were married.

When she arrived home unexpectedly later that morning, she told her mother she had come from school because she had a migraine headache. That way, her mom wouldn't ask a lot of questions.

The aftermath

As she lay in bed, Valerie began to experience severe cramps, worse than she had ever had before. But she had such a feeling of relief about being released from her pregnancy that she felt she could endure some physical reaction. Then she began to cry. She wasn't sure why she was crying, but she started to sob uncontrollably. She cried so hard that she had to bury her face in her pillow to muffle the sound. She didn't want her parents to hear her deep sobs.

That night Valerie kept waking up to find herself crying. In fact, she did not sleep well for many nights. These crying spells would hit her at different times. She would feel depressed and guilt ridden about having had the abortion. Then she would deny that the crying spells had any connection with that unpleasant experience.

Her feelings for Bill were changing. Deep inside she felt anger and resentment toward him for putting her through this whole frightening experience. After all, if he hadn't pushed her into sex, she would never have gotten pregnant. She resented the fact that he encouraged the abortion when he should have tried to stop her. She wondered if she could trust him. Did he really love her like he kept insisting? Would he look for the easy way out of other situations?

They began to have arguments and misunderstandings. He wanted to continue the sexual involvement. When she said, "No, I don't want to risk another pregnancy," he became hurt, angry, and demanding.

Postabortion grief

When they finally broke off their relationship and decided to date others, Valerie became so depressed that she couldn't keep her mind on school. She withdrew from her friends and would spend hours alone in her room. (Some girls have the opposite reaction. They are constantly looking for excitement because they cannot stand to be alone with their thoughts and feelings.) Valerie felt as if someone had died. In fact, she experienced the same feelings of grief that she had gone through when the family dog died two years before, only this was much worse.

For a while she wondered if she were losing her mind. She had terrible nightmares and began sleeping with a light on. After several months Valerie gradually began to recover, but she says that even now, after three years, she is still plagued by guilt.

Although she dates, she is afraid to get too close in a relationship with a guy. She also worries about marriage. She is afraid that her abortion will affect her relationship with a husband. What if he holds it against her? What if she can't have children? Will she be able to have a normal, guilt-free physical relationship with her husband?

What if a girl finds herself in a situation similar to Valerie's? Where could she turn for help?

Most cities now have prolife organizations, such as Physicians for Life, listed in the Yellow Pages under Abortion Alternatives Information. If a girl lives in a small town she can call the nearest office of the American Medical Association and ask for the names of several local prolife physicians. She might call her state capitol or the Health Department in her city for a listing of prolife organizations.

These are some Christian crisis pregnancy centers:

Auburne Center
7701 Belair Rd.
Baltimore, MD 21236
800-492-5530

Bethany Christian
  Services
901 Eastern, NE
Grand Rapids, MI 49503
800-BETHANY

Birthright International
686 N. Broad Street
Woodbury, NJ 08096
800-848-LOVE

Liberty Godparent
  Foundation
P.O. Box 27000
Lynchburg, VA 24506
800-542-4453

Christian Action Council
701 W. Broad St., #405
Falls Church, VA 22046
703-237-2100

Pearson Foundation
3663 Lindell Blvd., Ste. 290
St. Louis, MO 63108
800-633-2252, Ext. 700

Having the Baby

Fourteen-year-old Sharon said through her tears, "I hate being pregnant. I get sick every morning. It's embarrassing to be seen by my friends, and the boys in my neighborhood always have cute remarks or suggestive comments.

"My boyfriend left as soon as he found out I was pregnant. My parents have gotten so strict that I have to sneak around to go anywhere. I still want to go out with guys, but my parents say it's not right for me to be dating when I'm pregnant. I sort of understand, because it seems like every guy who takes me out just wants sex. I feel the only reason they like me is that they want to use me.

"I was supposed to start the ninth grade this fall, but it looks like I will have to wait till next year. That means I won't be in the same grade with all my friends. Oh, well, they have all pulled away from me, anyhow. They make me feel like I've got some kind of plague or something.

"How will I ever finish high school with a baby at home? I was thinking the other day that in ten years I'll be twenty-four and my baby will be ten.

"Oh, I hate being pregnant! My mom says I'll get stretch marks like she has, and I'll put on weight that I won't be able to get rid of.

"What guy would ever want to marry a girl who already has a baby? I hate being pregnant!"

One study reported that only half of the girls who give birth before age eighteen complete high school. On average, they earn half as much money and are more likely to be enrolled on welfare budgets: 71 percent of women under age thirty who receive Aid to Families with Dependent Children (AFDC) had their first child as a teenager. It's not easy, growing up in a welfare family. Medical care is usually substandard and inadequate. Family stability is often lacking. Impoverished neighborhoods are commonly crime ridden, and therefore moral values are routinely distorted.

The Rejected Child

One young, single mother recently told me that she simply didn't want her baby. She said, "I know I shouldn't, but I blame the baby for my losing my boy friend. It is not the baby's fault, but I just can't help feeling this way."

Will this attitude in the mother have any effect on the baby? Medical experts say that a baby can sense rejection right from birth. In fact, some recent studies indicate that even in the womb a baby responds to its mother's emotional reactions.

Angie, a young wife, said that her husband is working

two jobs, which seems to keep him tense and irritable. He comes home from his day job at 4:30 and leaves for his evening job at 6:00. There is always a lot of tension and bickering between them while he is home.

When she was pregnant, she noticed that the baby in her womb would get restless during the hour and a half each day that her husband was home. After the baby was born, he was fussy every day from 4:30 until 6:00.

Are births to unmarried teens any higher than they used to be? According to Chicago's National Opinion Research Center, in 1950 fewer than 15 percent of teenage mothers were single. By 1985 more than half (58 percent) and in some U.S. cities more than 75 percent were single.

The large majority of babies born to teenage single mothers are resented by their mothers. Such babies and young children often become the victims of abuse as they get older. Many young mothers cannot handle the constant pressure and responsibility of having to care for a young child twenty-four hours a day, 365 days a year, with no time off for summer vacation or holidays.

A Better Way

Rolly and Sandy, a young couple married for several years, had been unable to have a baby. They saw other couples having children and wondered why they couldn't. They felt frustrated and disappointed. Sandy said sometimes when other couples had a second and third child, she would cry out to God, "Why do they have several, and we have none?"

After seven years they learned that she was pregnant, and were they ever excited! They had so much fun preparing for the arrival of the baby they could hardly contain themselves. They spent every spare minute getting a bedroom ready, painting a dresser, buying a rocker, and stocking up on diapers for the arrival of this new family member.

Rolly said, "I'm not sure I believed we were actually going to have a baby until she was there."

When Sandy and Lesa came home from the hospital, there was a big sign on the house that read, "Welcome home!" The first meal they had together was a special celebration that included some other family members. When Rolly prayed at the meal, he cried as he thanked God for giving them Lesa.

Often, when Sandy went to put Lesa in her crib at night, she would pull back the covers and find a note from Rolly, which read, "I love you Lesa, and I love Lesa's mommy, too."

They seldom left her with a baby-sitter, because they wanted her with them wherever they went. In fact, Rolly sometimes took her with him to his office when he went to work.

They told me they feel perpetual thankfulness to God for the privilege of having a child.

Shouldn't the birth of a baby always be a beautiful event?

5

More Consequences of Messing Around
Sexually Transmitted Diseases

We've talked about a major consequence of messing around: pregnancy. Now let's move on to more consequences, those that might appear on the surface to be less life-changing but in reality may cause a lifetime of heartache.

Safe Sex?

One college guy asked me, "What about 'safe sex'? Most authorities are saying that's the way to keep from getting one of these sexually transmitted diseases."

That's a misconception I'd like to blast immediately. The surest protection against STD is abstaining from any premarital sexual activity. If you choose not to abstain, you need to know that your partner has not and is not engaging in any high-risk sexual activities that might have led to contracting an STD. There's a problem here, because in my experience I have observed that virtually everyone is unwilling to be totally open and honest with a current sex partner about the number and frequency of previous sexual encounters.

If you use condoms to prevent STD, you need to know that 10 to 20 percent of them have manufacturing defects. You must use them, preferably with a contraceptive foam, *every* time you have intercourse. Every time, without exception.

Given the discipline level of most high school and college students and their view of using condoms mostly as a means of birth control rather than disease prevention, it is easy to believe that they will not be using condoms each time they are sexually active. In fact, a recent study by the Alan Guttmacher Institute revealed that only 5 percent of sexually active persons aged fifteen to nineteen regularly used condoms.

Remember, there is no sure-fire protection against STD apart from abstinence. Our government, the medical community, and private business is spending billions of dollars in research and education in an attempt to stop the spread of STD. But not one of them is striking at the heart of the matter. They are not giving attention to the moral issues involved in the epidemic of STD. They do not refer to God's commandments. When people disregard God's principles, they open themselves to all kinds of attacks: spiritual, emotional, psychological, and even physical.

An Ever-Increasing Risk

If you mess around on the biological hand grenade ladder you run a very high risk of getting a sexually transmitted disease (STD). The Centers for Disease Control estimate that this year 14 million Americans will become infected with a sexually transmitted disease other than AIDS. That means that 38,000 people each day will become infected, or that *one out of four Americans will eventually be infected with an STD.*

The March 8, 1990 issue of *New York Times* reported that

Diseases like chlamydia, a pelvic inflammation suffered by women, and human papilloma virus or genital warts, have been at epidemic levels at many colleges in the last few years.

Two of every 1,000 college students has AIDS virus present in their blood, according to a government study done in 1989. "Okay, that's one in 500," said Dr. Henry W. Buck, chairman of the human papilloma virus task force for the American College Health Association. "What I tell college groups is that there is every reason to believe that the risk of human papilloma virus is one in ten. The risk for chlamydia is also about one in ten."

In other words, though the risk of AIDS is high, the risk of getting other STDs is many times greater. Although most high school and college students today are familiar with the AIDS crisis, many have never heard of the majority of these other diseases. But experts predict at least twenty-five STDs infect millions each year. And the victims are primarily teenagers and young adults.

When you ignore or disobey God's commands about sexual immorality, you not only set yourself up for the consequences of your sin, but you may also be subjecting your children to those consequences, too. Several sexually transmitted diseases can be transmitted from mother to child before, during, or immediately after birth, causing severe illness, deformity, and even death. In the January 30, 1989, issue of *TIME* (p. 69) it was reported that some 7,000 STD-related deaths occur each year in the United States, many of them in infants born to infected mothers.

God warns us about this in Exodus 20:5-6:

> For I, the LORD thy God am a jealous God, visiting the iniquity of the fathers [parents] upon the children unto the third and fourth generation of them that hate me; and shewing mercy unto thousands of them that love me, and keep my commandments.

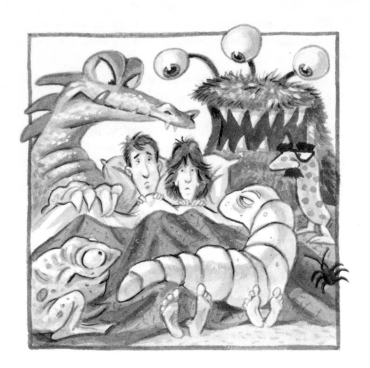

The Cost Runs High

The baby was, without question, the cutest one in the hospital nursery. At least that's what Jeff told everyone when he announced the arrival of his long-awaited daughter. He and Karen had been married eight years and had actually given up hope of having children.

Karen wasn't sure she wanted a child. She and Jeff hadn't been getting along well for a couple of years. She was becoming dissatisfied with her marriage but she kept hoping things would change.

Baby Kelly seemed to pull Jeff and Karen together. They both began to feel this may be what had been missing.

Kelly developed an eye infection. The doctor prescribed treatment, but before it was cleared up, the baby became sick with pneumonia. There was a period of panic, apprehension, and struggle to save the baby; but she recovered.

The doctor examined Karen and told her that the eye infection and pneumonia in her baby were caused by a sexually transmitted disease called nongonococcal urethritis. She was shocked. She didn't know she had an STD. Yes, it was true that she had had an affair, but she had broken it off shortly before she became pregnant. And she didn't have any symptoms to indicate a problem.

How Many STDs Exist?

The National Institutes of Health says there are over thirty known sexually transmitted diseases. We hear only about the worst and most prevalent ones.

In the introduction to a government study of sexually transmitted diseases, Dr. Paul J. Weisner says: "[lest we] become preoccupied with abstract numbers and . . . forget the human suffering caused by STDs, consider the teenage girl with genital herpes whose future is ravaged by recurrent diseases, who lives with the nagging fear of cancer, and who wonders whether her babies will be healthy. Or the young woman whose pelvic abscess is 'cured' by a total abdominal hysterectomy, who is robbed of future motherhood and is dependent on hormone replacement for the rest of her life. Or the young man who never heard of sexually transmitted hepatitis B until his liver biopsy showed the chronic active form of the disease."

The government estimates that each year well over fourteen million Americans visit their doctor or a clinic with an STD.

Some teenagers might respond, "So what, man? I don't know anyone with a sexual disease."

And to that I say, That's just it. You don't *know* anyone who has a sexual disease, either because they don't say anything or because *they don't even know* themselves. But, as you can see, studies show that these diseases are so common and widespread that, if you climb the biological hand grenade ladder with someone who has had other partners the question no longer is *if* you contract an STD; it is rather a question of *when*.

Gonorrhea

Gonorrhea is the second most common bacterial STD in the United States. Approximately 1.6 million cases of gonorrhea are reported each year. Although the number of reported cases has declined the past several years, they have declined more slowly among teenagers. *The Journal of the American Medical Association* (23 February 1990, 263:8, p. 1057) reports a tremendous increase in cases of penicillin-resistant gonorrhea infections. That means if you contract this bacterial infection, it might be very difficult to treat.

Jim and Debbie had been married for three years and had been trying to begin a family. Debbie had undergone medical tests that determined she was physically able to become pregnant. After much pleading on her part, Jim finally went to his doctor. He learned that he had become sterile due to a case of gonorrhea he had contracted as a teenager.

Jim had never told Debbie about his premarital sexual involvement. He had been treated for the disease at the time he contracted it and assumed that it would never be a problem. Now he wondered if she would ever trust him again since he had harbored this secret. Would she spend the rest of her life with him now that she knew he could never father the children she had always wanted?

In addition to inflicting excruciating pain on its victim, gonorrhea often causes sterility in women and sometimes in men. However, many women and even some men have no noticeable symptoms of early infection. This means that you could contract the disease and unknowingly pass it on until it causes a related problem later in life.

Syphilis

People in eighteenth-century Europe were dying like flies and filling insane asylums due to syphilis. This is a progressive disease which, if not treated, can cause brain damage, severe mental disorders, blindness, and eventually death. Even though a cure was discovered in this century, it is still a very serious problem, with an estimated over 325,000 *untreated* cases in America in 1988. According to 1990 statistics, the syphilis rate for teens (ages fifteen through nineteen) has increased by 67 percent since 1985.

Genital Herpes

By now most of us have heard of herpes simplex II, or genital herpes. But it has been widespread for only a few years. The first time Bob Palmer counseled someone who had contracted it was in 1977. This is a synopsis of the case history:

> The phone call came from the new husband just three months after they were married. I had spent several weeks with them in premarital counseling, trying to help them lay the foundation for a successful marriage. Now he was calling to say that since I had invested so much in the marriage, he thought I would want to know that he was filing for divorce.
>
> We agreed to meet and discuss the reasons for the divorce. When we met the next day, this new husband looked at me with pain and disappointment in his eyes and said simply, "She has herpes." He went on to say that while herpes is somewhat controllable, it is incurable, and he wanted to avoid contracting it because it can be very painful. He didn't want to continue to have sex with his wife, and could see no alternative to divorce. Not only this, but he was also heartsick to learn that his wife had previously had sex with another man, though she had given her

husband the impression he was the first and only one. This man told me his wife was in such pain from the herpes lesions (sores) at times, she could hardly walk. When she urinated, the pain was so intense she would scream and cry.

Genital herpes can be passed on to another person through sex even though there are no visible sores or apparent symptoms. Some babies contract genital herpes from their mothers at birth, and that about half of them will die as a result. Only 10 percent of the survivors will be normal.

National reports tell us that genital herpes has reached epidemic proportions, having affected an estimated 40 million Americans, and about 500,000 new cases will occur each year. At this point a herpes infection lasts a lifetime. There is no cure.

Genital Warts

My wife is a surgical nurse in a large metropolitan hospital. She is seeing an alarming increase in the number of patients coming in for treatment of condyloma caused by human papilloma virus (HPV), commonly called "genital warts" or "venereal warts."

You haven't heard of genital warts? You're not alone; many people haven't. However, studies show that in some areas the incidence of genital warts greatly exceeds genital herpes.

Already in 1985 Roy Rivenberg issued this warning in an article in *Focus on the Family* (p.3):

> Women with sexually transmitted disease face an increased likelihood of developing cancer. Herpes victims quadruple their susceptibility to cervical malignancies. And those who suffer from venereal warts are susceptible to cancer of the cervix and, occasionally among men, the penis.

These warts are not always visible to the naked eye but can be removed surgically or with lasers, chemicals, or liquid nitrogen. However, the virus cannot be cured.

Condyloma, like so many other STDs, is also on the rise in the United States, infecting approximately one million people each year.

Chlamydia

Chlamydia, an infection caused by the most common sexually transmitted microorganism in the United States, claims many victims. Experts estimate that over four million Americans develop a new chlamydia infection each year. About 40 percent of sexually active single women included in a recent study had positive blood tests for the antibodies to chlamydia. This indicates that they are either currently or previously were infected.

The majority of people who are infected with this insidious bacterial infection are totally unaware of it. Because it is symptomless, 70 percent of carriers have no indication of its presence or of the damage it is inflicting on them. Chlamydia silently causes major damage to the reproductive organs. It can impose major liver damage if it is not treated.

AIDS

AIDS (Acquired Immune Deficiency Syndrome), a fatal disease that according to the March 1990 issue of *Journal of the American Medical Association* claimed nearly 10,000 lives and struck 32,000 new victims in 1988 and over 35,000 in 1989, has currently infected about one million persons in the United States.

This disease is spread primarily by the exchange of body fluids which carry the HIV virus: blood, blood products, and semen (and possibly saliva and even tears). The principal means of transmission of the HIV virus is through any kind of sexual contact including genital, oral, and even French kissing. It is also spread by sharing contaminated I.V. needles.

Studies indicate that persons who have genital sores, syphilis, or herpes are at even greater risk of becoming infected.

Because of the controversy among experts on the size of the AIDS epidemic, many young people are being lulled into lethargy and carelessness. A report from the National Centers for Disease Control released in early 1990 estimated that the size of the AIDS epidemic was significantly smaller than originally projected. The CDC report stated that the earlier estimates, "based upon limited data available at the time, were too high."

Then in the March 16, 1990 issue of *Journal of the American Medical Association* (263:11, p. 1538), it was reported that the CDC stated,

> The observed incidence [of AIDS] in 1987 and 1988 exceeds projections. Data from HIV . . . surveys indicate that perhaps 1 million people have been infected. . . . If this is so . . . then the estimate of 200,000 cases will fall seriously short.

Studies indicate that AIDS is doubling every 2.8 years. Experts say teenagers are especially at risk because they usually have more than one sexual partner and very few teenagers use condoms. One in 200 teenagers who graduate from high school in Washington, D.C., is infected with HIV. A leading infectious disease expert has estimated that in ten years one in 200 males and one in 400 females in America will be HIV positive.

It is already distressingly prevalent in colleges. The *American Medical Association News* (2 June 1990, p. 24) related that two of every 1000 college students tested positive for HIV.

Because a person can carry the HIV virus for many

years without obvious symptoms and because there is neither a cure for AIDS nor a preventive vaccine, it will continue spreading quietly and rapidly among sexually active people.

According to Joe S. McIlhaney, Jr., in *Sexuality and Sexually Transmitted Diseases* (Baker, 1990, p. 149)

> There is no "safe sex" when one partner has AIDS. In one study it was found that when couples had intercourse without protection, thirteen out of sixteen uninfected partners became infected. If couples used condoms, two out of twelve (17 percent) became infected during the short period of the study. And these were couples in which the uninfected partner knew that his/her partner had AIDS and was being excruciatingly careful about using so-called protective measures.

But as I consider these statistics, I am again reminded of God's plan. God says to refrain from sex until there is a commitment to a faithful, monogamous relationship built on trust. Isn't that what these doctors are also suggesting? The only difference is they usually are not relating it directly to marriage as the Lord does.

6

Hidden Consequences of Messing Around

The most obvious consequences of premarital sex are unwanted pregnancy and sexually transmitted diseases. But there are others.

Loss of Virginity

The initial consequence of messing around is the loss of a person's virginity. However, the loss of her virginity is not simply a physical result for a girl. It has a far-reaching impact mentally, emotionally, and spiritually. Nor is virginity limited to girls; it is also important for guys.

For a girl, her virginity is not something she "loses" but rather something very personal and very sacred she gives away. It is not just having sexual relations for the first time or the breaking of her hymen. It is the giving of her total self, that which is to be given exclusively to one man for the development of a uniquely intimate relationship. A girl can give her virginity away only once in her entire life. This is true for a guy as well, for when two people engage in sexual intercourse, they give something of their whole being which cannot be recalled.

Now, you may be thinking, *Aw, c'mon, Bob, what is this, an instant replay of the Dark Ages? Don't you know that things have changed? Nobody waits until marriage for sex anymore.*

Look at what God says in 1 Thessalonians 4:3–6 (PHILLIPS):

> God's plan is to make you holy [Can you believe that? It is really true. God plans to make you holy.], and that entails first of all [Notice where God begins: "first of all"] a clean cut with sexual immorality. Every one of you should learn to control his body [Did you catch that? We have to learn to control our bodies, which means control that is not automatic. We will face temptations where we will have to learn to control our bodies], keeping it pure and treating it with respect and never regarding it as an instrument for self-gratification, as do pagans with no knowledge of God. You cannot break this rule without in some way cheating your fellow men [your partner and your future mate]. And you must remember that God will punish all who do offend in this matter.

That last sentence is true, but don't get hung up on it. There is complete and unconditional forgiveness found in Jesus Christ.

Emotional Consequences

Larry was a student in a Bible college. The first time he dated Cynthia, she snuggled right up to him in the car and put her arm around him some of the time while he was driving. He couldn't believe the woman, she was so aggressive. When he took her home, she suggested they park half a block from her house so they could "sit and talk."

She subtly but aggressively led him into a heavy necking session. Not that he minded. He enjoyed it.

By the third or fourth date, she had not only allowed it but had also encouraged Larry into sexual involvement. Every time they went out, they would wind up having intercourse. Strangely, Larry really didn't like Cynthia. The only reason he continued to date her was for sex.

Then one day, the thing he feared most happened. Cynthia's period was late. After she told him, he was a nervous wreck. When he told me about it, he said, "I'll tell you one thing, Bob, I'm not marrying that 'alley cat.' I don't even like her. But, what in the world am I going to do? I could join the army. I could transfer to a college at the other end of the country. I can't sleep nights. I can't enjoy anything."

Later, when I talked with Cynthia, she was going through the same mental anguish. A hundred times a day she wondered, Am I or not? Am I or not?

Possible suicide

Pregnancy is reported to be the most prevalent reason for suicide among teenage girls. And suicide is the second greatest killer of teenagers.

I have been at two different youth conventions where a girl tried to commit suicide because she was afraid she might be pregnant.

Nagging memories

Then there is the nagging memory, the inability to forget. This can come at you from two directions. One is the shame you feel when you remember your sexual experiences. You wish you could erase them from your mind, but you can't. The memories are imbedded there.

From the other direction, those memories are stirring up lust. If you relive past experiences in your mind, your fantasizing will re-ignite those powerful, lustful desires.

Unreasonable comparisons

Sherry had been married to Frank only a few weeks when she came to my office to talk about her marriage.

Frank had "slept around" with a number of girls before he met Sherry. He was constantly comparing her with the others. She was feeling rejected, unloved, unappreciated, and inadequate.

Girls may not fully realize that because males are so sexually oriented in their minds, they might constantly compare their partner's performances, body, and responses to those of other women they have taken to bed.

Remember, you are undermining your own marriage by getting sexually involved prior to marriage.

Preoccupation with sex

You can develop a distorted view of sex by becoming preoccupied with it. Guys especially get caught in this trap of sexual preoccupation.

The attitude of some guys is, "Hey, let's go get it. It's out there just waiting. Man, it sure feels good, and it makes me feel good, like I really am somebody."

Notice the selfish, self-centered outlook there. It is all "me, my, and I." That is why some guys can go out and pick up absolutely any girl who is willing to go out with them. They will take her out for sexual intercourse, just as they would take her out for a hamburger and shake, and drop her off with no thought for her feelings. Then they head out for ball practice or work, having satisfied their sexual appetites, just as they would their appetites for food.

To use and discard a human being certainly does not reflect a godly view of a person's worth, does it?

Daily suspicions

Distrust is another consequence of premarital sex. It will plant seeds of distrust between two people that may not bear fruit for several years.

Rick and Cynthia had been married nearly twenty years when they came for counseling. She had already filed for divorce because he had been abusive and she was afraid to continue living with him.

She said she had never felt fulfilled in their sexual relationship. He never seemed to consider her feelings. He seemed only to think about himself.

Rick said he felt as though she never really gave herself fully to him or to their relationship. He said, "We had premarital sex and I don't think we ever got over the effects of that."

"You're right," Cynthia responded. Turning to me she continued, "I felt so guilty. I had asked him to wait until we were married but he kept pressuring me. Immediately after I gave in, I was sorry.

"We have never discussed it or prayed about it or sought God's forgiveness. This is the first time since it happened, twenty years ago, that it has ever been mentioned, and I think it has contributed to the disintegration of our marriage."

When the honeymoon is over and the marriage just becomes "daily," she wonders what he is doing when he is away from her. He wonders whom she is talking to behind his back.

Either of them may begin thinking, Hey, if we messed around before we got married, is this marriage bond some kind of guarantee? Is it a wall—an invincible wall that no one can come over or under or through, and no one within the wall goes out? Or does it have weak places in it?

Social Consequences

Loss of respect

"How did you feel about your youth pastor after he had become involved in an affair with you?" I asked one young woman.

"I lost respect for him, Bob. I used to think he was the greatest example of a Christian I had ever known. When he first began to show an interest in me, I was flattered.

Then, when I realized it was a romantic interest, I was elated. It made me feel like I was the most attractive, special girl in the church.

"As the relationship grew, I began to realize that all he wanted from me was sex. He didn't really care about my feelings or about me as a person, just my female sexuality. That's when my respect for him began to die. I lost respect for myself, too. To think that I would do such a terrible thing. After all, he was married and had two children. I really liked his wife, and I began to think about how hurt she would be if she ever found out about our affair.

"Some of my friends began to suspect what was going on, and they lost respect for both of us."

Yes, loss of self-respect, mutual respect between you and your partner, and the respect of others are all at stake.

Parental pain

Now, the really "heavy one" is the pain in telling your parents about your sexual involvement, particularly if it has resulted in pregnancy.

Because of her attitude, her mother forced her to come to see me every Friday for four weeks. Her mother would wait in another room while we talked.

She was fifteen years old, and I could tell by the look on her face that she didn't want to see me that first time. At the end of the session, I said to her, "I have discovered something. There are two things that usually go hand-in-hand with something else. Drinking or drugs, and sometimes both, usually go hand-in-hand with sex." I didn't know a thing about her but I had a "gut-level" feeling that I was close. I continued, "You can write it down: Drinking and drugs cause people to lose control. What they have believed disappears; their values go right down the drain, and their standards go out of the window."

When she came back the next week, she said, "Mr. Stone, I didn't want to be here last week."

"It was written all over your face," I said.

"One thing you said at the end of our time last week made me realize you knew what was going on," she admitted. "I'm waiting for the doctor's report, and I have missed two periods already."

"So, what are you going to do?" I asked.

"I'm going to run away."

"Oh, that would be great," I responded.

After talking for a while, she realized that it was better to tell her parents personally than to have them find out through a call from the doctor's office. She was afraid to tell her father, because he had an explosive temper and she feared what he might do.

I asked her mother to come into the room. The fifteen-year-old daughter said, "Mom, I've got something very . . ."

She could not finish her sentence. She sat there in silence for what seemed at least ten minutes with a lump in her throat that must have felt as big as a baseball.

When she finally stammered out those stinging words, "Mom, I'm pregnant," her mother leaped out of the chair and lunged across the room toward her. I thought her mother was going to "belt" her. She bolted toward her daughter with both hands out, and for a moment I was ready to jump between them to keep her from beating her daughter. Instead, she put her hands around her daughter's head, pulled it to her shoulder, and said about fifteen times in a row, "Oh, I love you, I love you, I love you . . ."

As I watched the scene, it seemed I could almost hear that mother's heart deflate, just like a tire going flat.

Get ready to break some hearts, including your own, your partner's, and your parents', if you mess around on the biological hand grenade ladder. You can't build happiness on someone else's unhappiness.

I have a little saying that may help you to understand a basic difference between guys and girls: A guy thinks with his glands; a girl thinks with her soul. In other words, a guy can be so hung up on the physical relationship that he doesn't consider the feelings of others. He is hungry to have his physical appetite satisfied.

A girl, on the other hand, is more apt to control her physical desires. She is concerned not only about her feelings but also about the feelings of others who will be affected by what she does.

Do you think that while a guy is "getting his jollies" he is encouraging happiness in his girlfriend? No way. One girl said to me through her tears, "I was planning to be a missionary. Now I can't because I'm pregnant."

Damaged communication

Another consequence of premarital sexual involvement is the destruction of communication between the man and woman. Communication is more than just talking; it is sharing heart to heart. It is letting the other person look way down inside you, into your heart, to see what you are really like. It is exchanging not only what you think and how you feel about things, but also when and where you hurt and what makes you happy.

Why, then, is communication destroyed by premarital sex? I think there is one major reason.

When two Christian people are going together, God is very interested in their relationship, because he cares about each of them. The direction of their lives will be greatly affected, if not totally determined, by the person with whom they spend their lives. When the couple gives in to their natural, physical desires there is a great big cloud of guilt that settles over that relationship like a dense fog, not only between each of them and God, but also between the two of them.

Relationship Consequences

Relationship to God

I believe it is God's wish first of all that each of us develop a deep and meaningful relationship with him. Then he exhorts us to think not only about ourselves but also about other people and their welfare. "Each of you should look not only to your own interests, but also to the interests of others" (Phil. 2:4 NIV). This means not taking advantage of the other person or exploiting him or her for our own selfish desires.

Our first consideration should be to build our relationship on a foundation of spiritual unity before the physical relationship of marriage.

Relationship to each other

Christian couples engaging in premarital sex have gone against their consciences, for Christians know that love strives for the good of the other before the satisfying of self. Therefore, basic trust has been violated in their relationship. Now there is a wall keeping them from opening up to each other and being completely honest. The guy tends to become preoccupied with sex and is insensitive to the girl's feelings. And do you know where that cloud of guilt is resting? Usually on the woman, because she "thinks with her soul"—is preoccupied with feelings, heart-to-heart sharing, and commitment. So often a woman's love and sense of commitment runs deeper than a man's. A guy may feel guilty but will tend to rationalize the wrong he does, while a girl will draw a more clear-cut line between right and wrong.

A girl may feel it's not fair for her to have to carry this responsibility, but in most cases it is up to her to set the standard and draw the line on physical involvement. I agree with Dr. McIlhaney when he says (*Sexuality and Sexually Transmitted Disease*, p. 68, 69),

It is my opinion that womankind must resume the role they relinquished about thirty years go—that of setting the standards for sexual activity in the male/female relationship. I strongly urge you to avoid sex until you are married. If you are involved sexually with a man now, that relationship has a near 100 percent chance of breaking up. If and when it does, I highly recommend that you not get involved sexually with the next man you get close to until he marries you. Many men will avoid marital bonding as long as they can. If they can have what they want without assuming the obligations of marriage, a number of men will sidestep that commitment as long as they can.

Wayne said to me, "When my girlfriend and I got involved in a physical relationship, I actually felt my self-control slipping away. I want to be a godly man and had determined I would not give in to sex like so many of my friends. I know God wants me to be a man of convictions and a spiritual leader in our relationship, and my intention is to be that kind of man. But when we began to express our love through kissing and stuff, I actually felt myself being taken over by my desires. I sat there thinking, *We shouldn't be doing this, we've got to stop*. But I couldn't bring myself to do it. Becky had to be the one to say, *Stop*."

James 1:14 (NIV) talks about this: "but each one is tempted when, by his own evil desire, he is dragged away and enticed. Then, after desire has conceived, it gives birth to sin."

When a guy is in control of this area of his life, he not only gains the trust and respect of the girl, but he also grows in his spiritual maturity. Romans 6:19 (NIV) says, "Just as you used to offer the parts of your body in slavery to impurity and to ever-increasing wickedness, so now offer them in slavery to righteousness leading to holiness."

Spiritual Consequences

Guilt is not just a mental or relationship response, though. Guilt is also a function of a person's spirit. That is why some people are never able to get rid of guilt.

This brings us to a discussion of another group of consequences of premarital sex: spiritual consequences.

Lack of power

A "biggie" in this area of consequences is the loss of spiritual power in your life. Did you know that if you have invited Jesus Christ into your life, there is a supernatural power available to you? It far exceeds ordinary human power. This power is available to you for living the Christian life. You can't live it on your own, right? But Jesus Christ can live it through you.

Once you have tasted of something that powerful and then you lose that power, you are almost like a Samson who has had his hair cut off.

Loss of Christian fellowship

Young people who become deeply involved in sex are in danger of gradually losing their appetites for Christian fellowship and activities. They no longer want to be around spiritual events, Bible studies, or group discussions about the Christian life and keys to living it. No, they will avoid anything in a group setting that touches a personal nerve.

A negative advertisement

I couldn't figure out why one guy seemed so interested in Christianity yet wouldn't accept Christ.

This high school guy was six feet, two inches tall, weighed 205 pounds, and had muscles in places I don't even have places. He sat in the cafeteria with me for an hour and a half and listened as I explained how he could become a Christian. But he would not make a decision to invite Christ into his life.

Two years later, when he did become a Christian, I found out why he had put it off for so long. He had been going to bed with one of the girls in the group of which I was the leader. In his heart he felt they were being immoral, and because she called herself a Christian their relationship was a stumbling block to him. But we had faith that Christ would not give up on them, and he did not.

Your body, the temple

Is it wrong? Is sex outside of marriage really wrong?

First Corinthians 6:19–20 says that "your body is a temple of the Holy Spirit" (NIV). Do you think that God wants his temple endangered and defiled?

First Corinthians 6:18 tells us to "flee fornication." Don't just turn around and gracefully tippy-toe away in the other direction, don't trot, don't jog; sprint! Go with everything that is within you in the opposite direction. That's what God is saying to you.

First Peter 2:11: "abstain [stay away] from fleshly lusts."

Romans 13:14: "make not provision for the flesh, to fulfill the lusts thereof."

You often know what is coming, don't you, and you can plan those private times.

The NIV translates Romans 13:14, "do not think about how to gratify the desires of the sinful nature." God is cautioning us not to spend time figuring out ways to be alone in seclusion with a dating partner so we can pursue physical intimacy.

"I find myself constantly plotting ways to be alone with Heather," Chuck, a new Christian, told me. "I know good and well we'll end up in a heavy necking session and I'll be frustrated because I want things to go farther."

When I showed him this verse he was surprised. "I didn't know the Bible had such practical instruction," he commented. I guess it would be better to not dwell on those thoughts. That would probably cut down on my frustration level considerably. And obviously, it would be more pleasing to the Lord."

This is what it comes down to; you either want your way or God's.

If you are saying, "I'm not going to apply this to my life. I know I should, but I don't want to give up the pleasure, even if you think it will be rough later," I hope your attitude will soon become one of openness, of looking for answers. Otherwise, there is a lot of pain and destruction ahead for you.

7

How Far Is Too Far?

After I finished speaking to a group of high school kids, a girl walked up to me and said, "The way you talk, you make me think I shouldn't even let a guy hold my hand on a date. Are you suggesting we should have no physical contact until my fiancé takes my hand to put the engagement ring on it?"

"No," I said, "but there are a lot of things to consider about your dating relationships and the degree of physical contact involved."

One of the questions I asked in a survey of parents was, "As you study the rungs on the biological hand grenade ladder, ideally, where would you want your son or daughter to stop?"

Not one parent wanted a child to go beyond a light kiss. When asked why, all of them replied that once the lingering kisses begin, the participants are losing control of their emotions.

After discussing their standards and limits, one college couple decided they would confine their expressions of affection to an occasional hug. They knew that kissing would ignite emotions that would be difficult to control.

What, if anything, does God say about this?

"It is good for a man not to touch a woman" (1 Cor. 7:1).

After seeing that verse, one teenager said to me, "There, that proves it! God doesn't want us to have any fun if he really means what he says."

Why would the Bible make a statement like this? Well, let's consider some facts about touch.

"Touch is stronger than verbal or emotional contact. It affects nearly everything we do. It can produce the most sensuous pleasures, set off our deepest emotions," according to Diane Ackerman in an excerpt from her upcoming book, *A Natural History of the Senses,* which appeared in *Parade* magazine (25 March 1990, p. 5).

She goes on to say:

> Dr. Saul Schanberg, a professor of pharmacology and psychiatry at Duke University, believes: "Touch is far more essential than our other senses."
>
> Dr. Tiffany Field, a child psychologist at the University of Miami Medical School, says, "It's amazing how much information is communicable in a touch."
>
> "Touch affects the whole organism, as well as its culture and the individuals with whom it comes in contact. It's stronger than verbal or emotional contact," Dr. Schanberg explained, "and it affects (nearly) everything we do. No other sense can arouse you like touch. We always knew that, but we never realized that it was biologically driven.
>
> "If touch didn't feel good, there'd be no species, parenthood and survival," he adds. "A mother wouldn't touch her baby in the right way unless she felt pleasure doing it. If we didn't like the feel of touching and patting each other, we wouldn't have had sex."

Notice that Dr. Schanberg maintains that touching and patting are directly related to sex. And then look again at 1 Corinthians 7:1, "It is good for a man not to touch a woman." The Greek word translated "touch" literally means "to set on fire: kindle, light." So the verse is actually saying, "Don't light a sexual fire in a woman."

A nurse I know works for an obstetrician-gynecologist and frequently counsels unwed mothers and sexually active teenagers. She made the interesting observation that for most girls, just a touch—skin against skin—from a male they are attracted to arouses romantic and sexual desires.

God intended arousal of sensual desires for a married couple to enjoy in preparation for sexual intercourse. Therefore, if touching ignites that little fire and if touching is "far more essential than our other senses" as Dr. Schanberg states, then we can begin to see why God says it is good for a man not to touch a woman.

Since we all have a God-given need to be touched and we are designed to respond to touch, especially touches from an attractive member of the opposite sex, it is easy to see how we can quickly lose control of our emotions.

You might say to me, "Okay, in light of all this, where do you think I should draw the line on the biological hand grenade ladder?" I won't answer that. Nobody else can draw the line for you. You have to decide for yourself what your limits will be. Where you draw the line depends on what kind of person you are, what kind of person you really want to be, and what your relationship is with God.

I will, however, give you some guidelines that may help:

1. Don't pull up.
2. Don't pull down.
3. Don't unbutton.
4. Don't unzip.
5. Keep your hands to yourself. (It is well-nigh impossible to "make out" without using your hands.)
6. Keep your tongue in your own mouth.

A girl walked up to me in Cleveland, Ohio, after I had spoken and said, "Oh, Bob, I've never heard anyone talk like you talk."

"Well, how do I talk?" I asked.

"So straight. Good grief!" Then she began to cry.

When I asked her why she was crying, she said, "Because of what you had to say about French kissing."

"What are your views?" I asked.

"The problem is, I agree with you. But that is the only way I have kissed for six years. How in the world am I going to stop now?"

"Well," I said, "if you know the Jesus Christ who walked on the water, whose father parted the Red Sea and raised his son, Jesus, from the dead, then you have that same power available to you to do anything you should do."

How do you decide where the line should be for you? I was given some wise advice by a close friend when I was a freshman in college: "Treat your date the same way you would want your sister to be treated by the guys she dates."

In his book *Why Wait?* (San Bernardino, Calif.: Here's Life, 1982, p. 335), Josh McDowell quoted one Christian young person who wrote, "Abstinence is the best preventative. You cannot finish something you never start. Refraining from even nominal physical contact until permanent commitment has been made may be best for you."

Josh responded with this statement. "This is the standard I adopted before I married: I will treat a woman on a date the same way I want some other man to treat the woman I will someday marry. In other words, I decided ahead of time to act on dates in such a way that I would never be afraid of my wife meeting any of my former dates."

Sex is progressive. God has designed us so that one activity leads to the next, right? Sin is progressive, too. In fact, look at what God says about it in Romans 6:19 (NIV): "Just as you used to offer the parts of your body in slavery to impurity and ever-increasing wickedness, so now offer them in slavery to righteousness leading to holiness."

Did you catch the one about "impurity and *ever-*

increasing wickedness" (italics added)? One step does lead to the next. Sexual desire is not sinful, it is a God-given gift. But the misuse of sex in disobedience to God is sin. Because sex is so pleasurable, who wants to wait? Why deny yourself one of life's greatest pleasures when it is so easily available?

God says WAIT! because he wants you to enjoy sexual pleasure to its fullest. When you give in to your impulses, you rob yourself of the maximum benefits that are ahead for those who wait. And once you start down that road, it is nearly impossible to stop and put your emotions in reverse.

8

Date or Acquaintance Rape

Sarah enjoyed dating Ryan and going to school activities with him. He was a take-charge fellow who had a great sense of humor and made her feel special. There were a couple of things that bothered her, such as his habit of speeding and running stop signs, but she thought these were things he would eventually outgrow.

They had gone to a party and were on the way home when he stopped in a secluded spot. She enjoyed his kisses and tonight was no exception. But suddenly he began to pet. She asked him to stop, but he ignored her and continued. She pushed his hand away and said, "Please, *don't* do this." But he put his hand back and told her to relax and enjoy it. Then he was pulling at her clothes, trying to undress her. Now, thoroughly alarmed, she demanded that he stop, but he made some comment about her wanting this as much as he did.

She struggled, cried, pleaded with him to stop. But he ignored her. He became more forceful and was so strong that no matter how hard she tried, he overpowered her resistance.

When she continued to resist, he got very angry. He slapped her, and told her if she didn't stop fighting, he would hurt her seriously. This certainly wasn't the Ryan she thought she knew, even though they had been dating for several months.

She was petrified. Fear of serious harm engulfed her. She was afraid to fight, so she lay there and cried quietly.

As they drove home, she kept thinking, "I've got to take a shower. I just want to wash him off me and then I'll feel better." When she got home, she went directly to her room, relieved that her parents were already in their bedroom. She called out, "Mom, I'm home," as she went into the bathroom to shower. She turned the water as hot as she could tolerate and stood in it until it began to cool. But neither her tears nor the hot water could wash away the painful memory of the evening.

Rape is a traumatic experience for a girl because it is not just a physical invasion of her body but is also a violation of her soul, her mind, her emotions, and her very personhood. For a girl, sex is such a deeply personal experience that she wants to share it only with her beloved. And she wants to give it as an expression of deep love; not taken from her forcefully. When she is so brutally violated, her natural response, out of a sense of shame, is to keep it secret. She is embarrassed to have such a terrible thing happen to her. She does not report it, or even share it with a friend.

Date or acquaintance rape has become a major, serious crime among college and high school students in America. According to a report in the *Journal of American Medical Association*, there is a rape every six minutes in the United States. Rape, or attempted rape, is the most prevalent violent crime committed on campuses and involves about seventeen of every hundred college women each year.

Contrary to popular belief, those who commit rape and other sexual violence are frequently known by the victim. Very few rapes actually involve strangers. Over half of the victims were dating the attacker.

In many cities, all of the rape cases on police files involve acquaintance rape. In large metropolitan areas stranger rape does occur, but in the suburbs and smaller cities, date rape is most common.

Many Christian girls are caught off guard thinking there is no danger of being assaulted by guys they meet in church or through campus Christian organizations. Sadly, rape counselors report a high incidence of date rape even among active church attenders.

Contributing Factors

Contributing factors in date rape are the tendency for a girl to become comfortable with a guy she has dated for several months, coupled with a tendency for a guy to become more aggressive with a girl he knows well, thinking she is becoming interested in expressing her feelings toward him physically. As the relationship progresses and they become more responsive and less resistant to physical involvement, the guy may assume she is as interested in sex as he is. So he pressures her for it.

Often in an extended dating relationship, the level of intimacy increases. The couple may resist going beyond a certain point most of the time, but because dating relationships involve emotions, there are unpredictable variables. The extent to which physical involvement goes at any given time may be affected by such things as the time in the girl's monthly cycle, the emotional stresses they may have undergone at home or with their roommates recently, how each feels about the dating partner, and how much time they are spending together alone.

That's why I encourage every guy and girl to establish their limits before they go out on a date. When you are under the emotional pressure of passion and romance, realistic limits are difficult to set. Clearly explain what your standards are and indicate that you will not violate them. Base your limits on scriptural principles. Make it clear that the Bible is the foundation for your standards, and that you are accountable to God for your actions.

If during their dating relationship a couple has engaged in some petting, a guy may presume that the girl would enjoy sex but doesn't want to appear aggressive. Because she doesn't want to lose him, a girl may allow the limits of intimacy to be pushed away. He mistakenly assumes this is a signal that she is interested in having sex. Then when he presses for intercourse and she tries to stop short, he is so excited sexually that he refuses to stop. His emotions are out of control, so he forces intercourse even though the girl may be fighting, pleading, and crying.

The majority of girls do not report the attacker in this kind of assault. If the guy and girl are in high school, the assailants often go unidentified because the girl fears her parents' reaction, thinking they may blame her or criticize her choice of friends. College women are especially vulnerable because the victim knows the assailant's friends and roommates. She may feel that no one will believe this nice guy could rape a girl, so she does not report the attack. Some investigators estimate that less than 10 percent of acquaintance rapes are reported to authorities. They are convinced that rape has become so widespread in the United States that at least every third woman in America will experience rape or attempted rape during her lifetime. Disturbing statistics, to be sure, but even more alarming are the recent reports that in at least one major city, rape arrests have quadrupled among boys under thirteen years old.

Reactions

"The sexual assault controlled my entire life," one woman told me in counseling. "I couldn't get it out of my mind. I felt like I was having a continual nightmare day and night. I got to where I couldn't study or work because I was so depressed. I just wanted to stay at home in bed." She told me this five years after the attack. Even then she was still having deep emotional problems.

You might think the emotional repercussions in a girl would be lessened if she were raped by a guy she were dating, but research shows differently. The emotional consequences of sexual assault are the same if a woman explicitly thinks, "I'm being raped," or she thinks, "He seemed like a nice guy. Why is he forcing me to do this? Why won't he let me go? I'm scared and this is painful."

Acquaintance rapes usually take place late at night or in the early morning hours of the weekend, generally in the assailant's car or home, and they involve so much verbal and physical harassment and threats of violence that the victim will fear for her life.

One of the mistakes that many victims make is trying to pretend the rape never happened. They attempt to go on with their lives as if they were totally unaffected. But a woman's physical and mental health has been significantly jeopardized. Even if she will not admit it, she probably feels she has lost all control of her body, her actions, and her personal safety. Not telling anyone or soliciting help is a mistake.

As soon as possible a rape victim should call a person she can trust, such as her pastor, a pastoral counselor, her best friend, a family member, a doctor, a rape response center, or a hospital emergency room. Because she will be in a state of shock, she needs someone she can trust to help her think through her options.

A next step should be to seek medical help, not only for her own welfare (to check for tissue damage, to get treatment for possible exposure to sexually transmitted disease, and to prevent pregnancy) but also to gather evidence which may be used in court. She may not choose to prosecute her assailant, but if she takes steps to establish evidence she will have the option later.

A woman also needs to know that many victims experience what doctors call "post-traumatic stress syndrome," a delayed reaction to the experience which may come on them several years after the assault. Experts find that younger women and girls as well as elderly women have an especially difficult time in recovering.

In the days to years afterward, most (probably all) women who have been raped will continue to react to the trauma in predictable ways. This pattern is called rape trauma syndrome.

Initially a girl will feel paralyzed or numb. Then she will begin to withdraw from her feelings and even from her friends. But as she moves away from her ordeal, she will experience a return of the sense of helplessness and terror, the two major things she felt at the time of the attack. This will bring on interludes of acute anxiety accompanied by such symptoms as sweating, rapid breathing, and a fast heartbeat. She may find herself feeling terrified at night. And she will probably cringe at the thought of having sex.

In married women who are experiencing revulsion at the thought of engaging in marital sex, counselors often uncover rape trauma syndrome due to an assault which they experienced years earlier.

Doctors look for three stages in rape trauma syndrome:

First, if a woman keeps silent about her assault she may experience headaches, insomnia, nausea, depression, anxiety, nightmares, and/or constant uneasiness.

Second, after a few days she will become absorbed with her role in the event, trying to figure out what she did to cause it or if she could have prevented it.

Third, as with any experience involving grief, she will begin to reorganize her life; accept the reality of the event; and deal with her fears, her friends, and her attitude toward men and sex. Her major battlefield will be confronting her own anger. She must acknowledge it and deal with it so she can gain freedom from its bondage.

Self-Protection

What should a girl do if she is attacked by her date or other acquaintance?

1. Do everything you can to get away.
2. Resist.
3. Yell for help, but do not become hysterical and scream in a high-pitched voice. Resisting and yelling are often effective in stopping a rape, but some men are stimulated and aroused by a woman's screams.

Law enforcement agencies and rape response centers advise against trying to disable the would-be attacker in most cases. Alabama police officer Lt. Ralph Long, who instructs women in self-defense techniques, said, "It is extremely difficult, if not impossible, for a woman to disable a hostile, aggressive man. In addition to that, if she does not totally disable the assailant, but only injures him, it will increase her chances of being seriously injured because an angry rapist will only become more violent."

A study by Dr. Charlene Muehlenhard (*New York Times*, 29 August 1989, C-6) confirmed that one effective tactic to avoid date rape is that the woman should make clear early in the encounter that she is not interested in having sex. Other effective approaches were physical resistance, screaming, and claiming to have a venereal disease. But the most powerful tactic of all was the statement "This is rape and I'm calling the cops."

There are those rare occasions when a girl may be assaulted in the presence of others (for example, on a double date). If confronted with this situation, it may help to appeal to the other girl and her date. If the attack takes place in the presence of other guys, a girl should ask one of them to protect her. Look directly at the one guy you feel would be most responsive, call him by name, and say, "Please, help me."

Girls also need to be aware that some guys think a girl is just being coy if she says no when she is pressured for sex. Many guys think she really means yes when she says no. If a girl means no she should say no emphatically. There is a difference between no and "No, I'd rather you didn't." If a girl is not firm and definite in her refusal, a guy could easily take her to mean, "I'd rather not, but it's okay."

Male Attitudes

She owes it to me

Beth was thirty-eight years old. Her husband left her two years ago, and she was lonely and depressed. A man she met through her job had become a good friend and was very understanding and comforting when he learned of the breakdown of her marriage. One day he invited her to have dinner with him "just to talk and unburden your heart." She was so impressed with his sensitivity to her emotional pain, and because he was just a good friend, she accepted his invitation.

He took her to a luxurious restaurant, bought her an expensive dinner, and listened intently to her for over two hours. Later, when they arrived at her home, they were in the middle of an intense conversation, so she invited him in for coffee. As soon as they were inside and the door was closed he grabbed her and while trying to kiss her began tearing at her clothes. When she resisted, he said, "What do you mean, no? I spent a lot of money on you this evening and you owe it to me to have sex with me."

"I don't owe you a thing," she retorted. "I can pay my own expenses. Here's the money for my dinner. Goodbye."

Forty-three percent of the high school and college age men included in a 1979 California study said that by the fifth date it was acceptable for a man to force sex on a woman, and 39 percent of the men said it was acceptable if the man had spent a lot of money on her (*New York Times*, 29 August 1989, C-6).

A girl needs to know if her date has the attitude (which may not become apparent until they are in an isolated situation where he has the opportunity to become aggressive) that she owes him sexual favors if he has treated her with special attention. This is really a form of buying sexual favors—prostitution!

Some guys think it's manly to overpower a girl and force her to give in to their demands. Guys who grow up in violent families often have the attitude that it is normal to use force or violence to obtain whatever they want. Also, most guys who are inclined to rape believe women are subservient to men. Avoid dating a guy who has a macho attitude, one who behaves as though women are less important than men.

Dominance, hostility

Research discloses that some men can become sexually aroused while reading a story, not necessarily classified as pornographic, in which a woman is forced to have sex.

> Dr. Neil Malamuth, a psychologist at the University of California at Los Angeles, observed the reactions of men to stories depicting sexual incidents.
>
> "The men who were most likely to become aroused by a story in which a woman was forced to have sex despite protests tended to share other attitudes. One of these was the idea that dominance itself was a motive for sex; they agreed with statements like "I enjoy the conquest." Another is hostility toward women, as expressed in sentiments like "women irritate me a great deal more than they are aware of" (*New York Times* 29 August 1989, C-6).

Manipulation

One of the most difficult areas the victim of date rape has to deal with is the issue of trust. This is because the guy who raped her had spent enough time with her to gain her confidence. He probably treated her with enough thoughtfulness that she believed he really cared about her. Because she trusted this man enough to be alone with him and he so blatantly violated that trust as to make her fear for her life, it destroyed her ability to trust anyone.

Guys like this are skilled manipulators. They learn to control a girl by complimenting her and building her up so that she feels special, very attractive, and appreciated. Then at other times they may become verbally or physically abusive. However, they will later be apologetic and beg for forgiveness and another chance. Why do girls allow and/or respond to this kind of treatment? Many girls have such feelings of worthlessness they feel they deserve to be treated cruelly.

An eighteen-year-old counselee had dated several older, married men. They had treated her with a mixture of kindness and abusiveness. I asked her why she had continued in the relationships after the abusiveness began. She started to cry and said she was such a terrible person that she deserved to be treated that way.

Psychological rape

Some men are psychological rapists. They seem to enjoy building up a girl one minute and tearing her down the next, playing Ping Pong with her emotions. They learn how to flatter a girl who may be struggling with her self-worth and who feels she is not very attractive or personable. They seem to get some sort of egocentric pleasure out of being in control of another person's feelings.

A college girl told me she fell for a guy because he told her very convincingly that she was absolutely beautiful. Although she was an attractive girl, her parents had made it a point not to emphasize her physical beauty but rather to concentrate on her inner qualities.

When this guy came along and began to overwhelm her with compliments and admiration for her beauty, her heart melted and she fell in love. She knew this guy would not be the kind of man her family and friends would approve of or encourage her to date. But because he made her feel so special he was able to manipulate her into having sex. Her heart was later broken when she learned he was doing the same thing with other girls.

Interpreting sexual interest

Men tend to assume sexy dress and a flirtatious manner logically mean a desire for sex. In discussing the problems of overcoming temptation with many young men, I have repeatedly heard from them that "girls who dress sexy or girls who come on to a guy are obviously offering sex."

When it comes to female behavior, younger men especially tend to have difficulty discriminating between what is merely friendly and what indicates sexual interest. As previously mentioned, pornography promotes the idea that girls crave sex just as much as lust-controlled guys. Soap operas are notorious for communicating the message that acquaintance rape is really seducing a woman. A woman drinking, coming to a man's apartment, or wearing "sexy" clothes may seen by men as indicators that the woman is interested in sex. Even friendliness on the part of a girl may be interpreted by some guys as an indicator that she is interested in sex. "Not so," say many women.

Defining rape

"When men are asked if there is any likelihood they would force a woman to have sex against her will if they could get away with it, about half say they would," said Dr. Neil Malamuth, a psychologist at the University of California at Los Angeles. "But if you ask them if they would rape a woman if they knew they could get away with it, only about 15 percent say they would. Those who change their answers do not seem to realize that there is no difference between rape and forcing a woman to have sex against her will," Dr. Malamuth said. Many women also share the confusion and so may not realize that they have been raped (*New York Times*, 29 August 1989, C-1).

Guys, don't believe the Hollywood hype that when a girl resists, she is really asking for sex. The idea that you should use force and persist until the girl melts in your arms is absolutely false. The truth is, anything other than total consent and willing participation is rape. A girl will actually respect you more if you honor her wishes.

The law is unclouded on this matter: In all fifty states it is illegal to obtain sexual intercourse through force or coercion or through the threat of violence.

The law as stated in the Alabama statutes is typical:

> A male commits rape in the first degree if he engages in sexual intercourse with a female by physical force that over-comes earnest resistance or a threat, expressed or implied, that places her in fear of immediate death or serious physi-cal injury to herself or another person.

Rape, in the eyes of God, is as serious as murder (see Deut. 22:25-27). Guys forcing girls to submit to sexual aggression is not new. It is probably as old as humanity itself. That's obviously why God made the law very clear in Scripture.

Remember, anything other than total consent and will-ing participation is rape.

Social Attitudes

In movies, rock videos, and men's magazines our culture promotes violence and sexual aggression against women. There is even a computer game, very popular in college dorms, that depicts nudity and encourages the computer operator to carry out electronic sexual aggression. As a result of the media assault on the minds of teens and young adults, attitudes have changed about violence in general, but especially about sexual violence against girls.

A junior high school administrator described the response of the boys to an educational program depicting the devastating trauma of a rape victim. The reaction was laughter, joking, and ridiculing the idea that a girl would be adversely affected by forced sex.

Someone has said, "Music is the language of the soul." Music can move people to react in many different ways. And I'm convinced that current popular music is contributing to the problems of rape and violence in our nation. A song "I Want Action" has a line in it that says, *If I can't have her, I'll take her, and make her.* Slick Rick, a popular rapper, has an album titled "Treat Her Like a Prostitute." The group called Guns 'n Roses sings: *I used to love her but I had to kill her.*

Recovery

Rape is not an act of sex, it is an act of violence. Violence leaves a person with deep-seated feelings of anxiety and fear. These feelings are followed by shame and guilt. The girl feels guilty because she thinks she did something to cause the rape. Guilt brings with it shame.

A person doesn't want to face God when he or she feels ashamed. Though the guilt and shame a rape victim feels are not the result of her sin (they actually belong to the rapist), those feelings are there. Her guilt causes her to avoid God. The pain the victim has suffered was forced on her by a selfish and insensitive person. God is just the opposite. He doesn't force, he waits for us to ask for his help. Then he gently begins to heal us.

Healing always requires time. Time does not heal; God heals. But healing does take time. The deeper the wound, the longer the time required to heal the wound. Because rape so deeply wounds a woman, she will require a long time, often years, to recover.

Many women never actually recover because they have not found the source of recovery. Recovery begins with God. "He healeth the broken in heart, and bindeth up their wounds. He telleth the number of the stars; he calleth them all by their names. Great is our LORD, and of great power: his understanding is infinite" (Ps. 147:3-5).

Anger

Recovery begins with God, but concealed or denied anger prevents God's work in a person's heart. To begin recovery, one of the first things a rape victim must confront is her anger, a normal reaction to rape and part of the built-in defense mechanism given by God to help her protect herself. She will be angry with the attacker, she may be angry with herself, and even angry with God. She may be consumed with anger.

Anger itself is not wrong. God is sometimes angry and Jesus got angry on certain occasions. The issue is not the anger but what a person does with that anger. If a victim remains in a state of aroused anger, it becomes her destructive enemy. Anger, if left unattended, can turn to rage; it feeds resentment and bitterness, and bitterness will destroy a person.

As the victim begins to confront her anger, she needs to sort through it. At whom is she angry, and why? If she realizes she is angry at God for allowing this to happen, she must not let her emotions rule her feelings but apply the truth of Scripture to her life. She may have to go strictly on faith, believing what the Bible says and allowing truth to override her feelings. The rebuilding of her emotional and psychological stability is greatly affected by her ability to trust God.

As God begins to bring healing to her heart, her anger will gradually turn to disappointment and sorrow. She can then find solace in the Lord as he comforts and restores her. He will show her his ability to supply the strength she needs to endure the trial. And then he lovingly provides the healing. But if she suppresses and contains her anger, it will eat away at her like a cancer.

The victim, therefore, must acknowledge her anger and confess it to God. God knows she is angry, but he wants her to recognize it and confess it to him. First John 1:9 says: "If we confess our sins he is faithful and just to forgive us our sins and to cleanse us from all unrighteousness." In other words, the rape victim needs to acknowledge her anger toward her assailant and realize that it was rape, it was his fault, and the guilt belongs to him. She then can be free from guilt and shame.

Self-worth

Rape causes a woman to question her self-worth. She feels dirty and unworthy. She must come to see her worth to God, that she is valuable to him, and that he wants to comfort and heal her. She can turn to God and find comfort and peace in him.

Often a girl will ask, "Why did God allow this to happen to me?" Most of us ask that question when suffering and pain invade our lives. God did not promise to spare us from suffering. In fact, he warned us we would face trials. God may allow suffering to deepen a person's relationship with him, which in turn allows him to bring healing and comfort into that life.

Forgiveness

Resentment and bitterness are sins God warns against. They are a direct result of not forgiving. Jesus commanded us to forgive those who wrong us. And forgiving is essential to healing. "For if you forgive men when they sin against you, your heavenly Father will also forgive you. But if you do not forgive men their sins, your Father will not forgive your sins" (Matt. 6:14 NIV).

It will take time, perhaps several weeks or months, for a girl to be emotionally healed enough before she can even begin to think about forgiveness, but the time must come or she will never be totally free.

To really be free from the ever-present aftermath of rape, a girl must ask God to give her the grace to forgive the guy. And in the case of such a traumatic experience as rape, forgiveness is often a slow and growing process. The rape victim is not responsible for what has been done to her, but she is responsible for her response. If she wants to be healed, she must accept her responsibility to draw near to God for his strength and, with his help, forgive her offender.

Learning to trust again

One of the biggest challenges to the date rape survivor is learning to trust herself again, that is, to trust her judgment of people and circumstances. She misjudged her dating partner, so her self-confidence has been shattered. Consequently, she will be unsure of her decisions and evaluations in the future. She is not sure she trusts anyone, not even God. And if she can't trust God, whom can she trust?

The girl who is trying to recover from rape and struggling with her capacity to trust God will find real help in these books: *Why Us? When Bad Things Happen to God's People* by Warren W. Wiersbe (Old Tappan, N.J.: Fleming H. Revell, 1984) and *Where Is God When It Hurts?* by Philip Yancey (Grand Rapids, Mich.: Zondervan Publishing Co., 1977).

Exercise

One important key in recovery is physical exercise. Exercise helps a victim feel good about herself. She not only regains control of her body but also uses up energy that otherwise might be uselessly spent emotionally reviewing her experience. Being tired will also help her sleep better. The physical aspect is important because it is tangible. She can measure her progress, which will give her a regained sense of control and confidence to take charge of other areas of her life.

Exercise helps recovery from many forms of emotional trauma, especially depression. When a girl has been raped, depression is one of the major feelings she will battle. If we can get a person who is struggling with depression to establish a mild, daily exercise program with a minimum of twenty minutes of exercise a day, within two weeks the symptoms of depression begin to disappear.

Tell a trusted friend

One of the elements of recovery is to encourage a girl to confide in someone she trusts completely. *She must tell someone about the assault.* Most girls fear rejection, remain silent, and thus allow the problem to fester inside, often for years.

We have had countless women come for help with some problem that has troubled them deeply for a long time. Frequently as they open their hearts, an experience of sexual assault will surface and spill out along with their tears. Most of them will say this is the first time they have ever told another person.

God tells us to bear one another's burdens. A burden that heavy is too much to bear alone and must be shared. Opening up to another person nearly always has a healing effect.

Confronting the assailant

In date rape recovery counseling, many counselors encourage the victim to eventually confront the assailant to make him aware of the pain he has caused her and to vent her anger toward him. Although confrontation is a scriptural thing to do (Matt. 18:15), it should not be done to vent one's anger. The objective of confrontation is to help the Christian brother who is doing wrong and to restore fellowship between that person and the one who was wronged.

A girl's need for protection and security must be considered in asking the victim to confront her offender. Most rape survivors state emphatically that they never want to see the rapist again. They want to avoid further contact in any form.

The rapist should be confronted by another male, such as the victim's father or brother. She will find comfort in knowing that her offender has been exposed and confronted. This will help relieve her anger, begin rebuilding her sense of security, and reestablishing some trust in men.

Most guys who force sex on a girl they are dating are probably never confronted with what they have done to the girl and will probably go on to assault other girls. If the victim will ask for help and a male in her family will take the responsibility to confront the assailant, this may make him aware of the devastation he has caused and possibly prevent him from victimizing another unsuspecting girl.

Prevention

What steps can a girl take to keep herself safe from potential date rape?

1. Don't go out alone with a guy you don't know. Make plans to double date. But even then, go with someone you know. If you are the stranger in the group you may find yourself standing alone in a losing battle.

Cynthia went on a double date with Jim, his friend Ken, and Ken's girlfriend. She said she had never met the other couple so she had no idea they would be blatant about their sexual involvement. They began getting intimate during the date and Jim proceeded to pressure her. When she resisted, the other couple ridiculed her for being a prude. They did nothing to discourage Jim from forcing her into sex.

2. Determine ahead of time what your standards and limits are and state them explicitly to your date. Don't ignore a minor infraction of the rules. Remind him of the limits you have set. Keep reminding him each time he tries to bend them. Stay away from any guy who pokes fun of the agreed-to rules once you are out on a date with him.

3. Watch for danger signals. The guy who is prone to

date rape will often be aggressive and pushy. He will constantly try to touch you in an effort to make physical contact. Then he will suggest going to a place where the two of you can be alone. He is looking for isolation.

4. If anything he does makes you uncomfortable, say so at once. Don't be afraid to embarrass or offend him. A common saying among rape counselors is, "Better rude than raped."

5. Stay away from any place where drugs and alcohol are in use. Fifty percent of rapes are alcohol or drug related.

6. Don't give mixed messages. Don't say no with your mouth and yes with your body language. If he touches you in a place you do not want him to touch you, move his hand away firmly as you say stiffly, "Take your hands off me." Be outraged! Your body does not belong to him.

7. Listen to your instincts but do not rely exclusively on them. Your emotions can blur the message the instincts are trying to send. Or your instincts might be deceived. If you feel uncomfortable with the way a guy is treating you, or if he is making unreasonable demands or questionable requests, put an end to the relationship. Do not take risks.

Janet was nineteen and newly married. A few weeks after their wedding, the government sent her husband to Tokyo for three years. Because she would not be allowed to join him for six months, she decided to spend one semester at Eastern Michigan University in Ypsilanti, Michigan, taking advantage of the scholarship she had been awarded.

She told me her roommate was dating a student named John Collins, one of the nicest, most polite, and thoughtful young men she had ever met. Janet had many enjoyable conversations with John.

One day he asked her if she had ever ridden on a motorcycle. When she said no, he offered to take her for a ride. She wanted to go but hesitated because she was married. She thought it would be a lot of fun but didn't want to do anything that could be misunderstood by others. Though it would have been perfectly innocent, she knew it might appear to others that she was going out with another guy while her husband was away.

When she told John she couldn't go because she was married, he said, "Oh, come on, your husband is clear around the world. He'll never know."

"Maybe not," she responded, "but I'll know and so will the Lord. And besides, other people might take it wrong."

Six months later she joined Larry in Japan. When she received some newspapers from home, she eagerly began reading them. On the front page of one issue the headline announced that Eastern Michigan student John Collins had been arrested for the rape and murder of eight coeds. When she saw the headline she said, "This must be a mistake. John couldn't be the murderer. He is such a nice young man."

The article went on to say that his method of operation was to invite a girl for a ride on his motorcycle. He would take her to an isolated spot where he would assault and kill her.

Janet felt sure that if she had trusted only her instincts, she probably would have been victim number nine. But she obeyed God's Word and the prompting of his Holy Spirit by avoiding even the appearance of evil.

8. Be unusually alert during holidays that are especially significant for teens and young adults. Many pregnancies begin around spring break and special holidays such as July Fourth and Valentine's Day.

9. Remember the powerful tactic, the statement "This is rape, and I'm calling the cops." Although difficult for a girl with a compliant or nonassertive personality, if she wants to avoid date rape she should work at being direct and confident in her refusal to do anything she does not want to do. Studies show that typical victims of date rape were not good at asserting themselves and usually suffer from low self-worth. A victim who was raped at a campus party

did not yell for help *because she was afraid she'd embarrass the guy.*

10. If you find yourself being accosted, cry out to God for deliverance. The one thing he required of a girl in Deuteronomy 22:25–27 who was about to be raped was that she cry for help. A woman whom I counseled was attacked and feared for her life. When she cried out to God, the attacker suddenly stopped, and her life was spared.

A Word to Guys

I hope you are beginning to grasp the disastrous effects of rape on a girl. I don't know if there is anything a guy could experience that would be as devastating and harmful to him as rape is to a girl. Guys are not as easily plagued by fear and feelings of helplessness, so it is difficult, if not impossible, to empathize with the deep pain and resulting consequences in a girl's life.

To a guy, sex is more of an external pleasure that does not necessarily involve deep emotional feelings and commitment of his total self to the person with whom he is having relations. He may struggle with the guilt of having committed sin, but he will not feel violated and used.

A woman is never totally free of the aftereffects of rape. For a long time after the assault, a woman will experience what is called hypervigilance. She becomes overcautious and is apprehensive about everything she does and everywhere she goes fearing, she may be accosted again. Then as the hypervigilance subsides, she continues to struggle with trust. She is afraid to trust any man in any situation. Rape is a deeply personal invasion, a violation, of her personhood as well as her body.

The victim may believe she is losing her mind. She is trying to make some sense out of the experience but can't. She will never understand why this terrifying ordeal happened to her when she didn't want it to and did nothing to cause it.

Virtually every rape survivor at some time during the assault feared for her life, no matter who the assailant was—an acquaintance or a stranger. At some point during the attack she was terrified that she might die. Fear is one of a woman's most common frailties. I believe God designed a girl to need protection. So when she finds herself in a situation where she has no control and is being exploited rather than protected, a girl will be overwhelmed with fear.

Many guys have been led to believe that to prove their manhood they must "score" with a girl even if it means forcing her to have sex. In fact, some teens think it makes them more of a man if they have to overpower a girl and force her into sex. But real men never use any kind of physical force on a woman. Nearly any man can overpower most women. God did not design a woman's muscle structure like a man's. So it really proves nothing when a man defeats a woman in a contest of physical strength.

I believe that a real man controls himself and his desires and does not take advantage of others for his own selfish pleasure or in response to his lust.

What about the guy who is inclined to rape? What causes him to employ his strength to overpower a physically weaker person and use her in an insensitive act of violence? Usually an abusive person has been an abused person. Guys who are inclined to rape are usually guys who have been abused and felt rejected, in most cases by their fathers.

The man who abuses a woman has a very low opinion of himself. He suffers from a sense of rejection, feeling that he must prove that he really is somebody. I always encourage people like this to realize you don't have to "be somebody"—you already are. You are special to the Lord. He created you to have fellowship with him, and he has a special purpose for your life.

Rape response counselors identify three types of rapists:

the dominator, who has a low sense of self-worth; the intimidator, who has buried and seething anger; and the psychotic, who was himself severely abused. I believe there is one more factor, but first let's look at these three.

The dominator is the guy who feels a need to defeat others. It makes him feel powerful and important if he can conquer another person. He has a deep sense of inadequacy and feels a need to prove himself. This type of rapist is also referred to as a power rapist.

The intimidator is a very angry man. He has deep resentment and bitterness toward someone who has hurt him in the past. He carries the anger inside, and it explodes when his emotions rage out of control. He enjoys intimidating and frightening his victim because he relishes the feeling of revenge that comes over him when he is controlling them and their emotions.

The psychotic rapist is one who has a severe mental disorder, has withdrawn from reality, and will carry out bizarre torture or even death.

I believe there is one more factor to be considered, which seems to be often overlooked, and that is the problem of lust. If a guy has an uncontrolled sex drive or concupiscence, and he has been feeding his appetite with lustful thoughts so that he is aroused sufficiently, nothing will stop him from getting what he wants from this girl.

If you are a male and you are thinking, *Hey, I have some of those feelings and have experienced a background like one of those you have described. I wonder, do I need help?* By all means, seek help from a Christian counselor or your pastor or a Christian doctor. Those feelings are indicators that there is something going on inside you that needs to be addressed.

Maybe you are a guy who is not overwhelmed by any of these major problems but you are a normal, red-blooded, American male who struggles with controlling his sexual appetite, and you want to treat the girls you date with proper respect and care. You don't want any girl to ever feel that you are forcing her into doing anything she doesn't want to do. You never want a girl to feel that she is being threatened with rape or anything close to it.

Here are some suggestions that will help you avoid any misunderstanding in this area.

1. Pray together. At the start of the date, ask the Lord's blessing on the time together and commit to him that you will not do anything dishonoring to his name.

2. Make a verbal commitment to the girl's parent(s) that you will protect her and not allow anything to happen that would worry or concern them.

3. Most of the time, make it a point to not go places alone. Double date or group date. If most of your time is spent with others it is unlikely you will become sexually involved. If you do single date, stay away from secluded places such as your apartment or your car in an isolated location.

4. Establish your limits ahead of time and discuss them with your date. Make it clear to her that you will never pressure her to do anything she does not want to do. Let her know that you are a young man with godly principles and that you intend to live by them.

5. Never assume that a girl is interested in sex because she is dressed in a revealing way or because her body language seems to indicate that she is. And just because she seems to enjoy kissing or even petting, do not assume she is inviting you to have sex with her. Some girls have not learned that kissing and petting are natural steps toward intercourse, and that when a guy participates in such activities he is becoming aroused to the point that he will not want to stop.

6. Stop any activity immediately if the girl shows any resistance or expresses a desire not to continue.

7. Stay away from alcohol and drugs altogether. As mentioned earlier, these substances were contributing factors in at least 50 percent of the rapes.

8. One of the most effective aids to a guy in maintaining his moral character is accountability. Make yourself accountable to another Christian guy who will hold you responsible for all of your actions and activities and will pray with you and for you.

9. Be prepared to stand alone in a group. Determine now that you will not give in to pressure from your peers. Some guys have said they have participated in sex when they really didn't want to when pressured by peers, for instance at a party where others were having sex.

10. Be particularly careful on special days, such as holidays. It is easy to spend too much time together on such days. Emotions run higher during these special times. There is more temptation to get carried away in the emotion of the moment or event.

11. Stay away from the "heat." You know which situations cause more temptations for you than others, and you are responsible to the Lord for the things you allow to enter your life. If you go out with a girl whom you know to be a temptress, you are putting yourself in a situation God specifically says to avoid. "Flee youthful lusts" (2 Tim. 2:22).

Remember, a girl's body does not belong to you. If she's a Christian, her body doesn't even belong to her; it belongs to God. Her body is a temple of the Holy Spirit. Look at it as holy property and treat her that way. The same goes for your body.

Realize you could mess up your own life, some guy's future wife, and you could thereby start an epidemic that will affect not only her but also their children and grandchildren.

A woman counselor told me that both her mother and grandmother had been sexually abused. Her grandmother had a bitter attitude toward men and had told her mother to stay away from men because they were "no good." Her mother was then raped and bore her at age thirteen. As a result, both of them had discouraged her from having anything to do with men. She was in college when she met a man who treated her with such godly love and kindness she fell in love and married him. Yet, after twenty years of marriage, she is still struggling to overcome the results of the pain inflicted on her mother and grandmother.

You can't build your happiness on someone else's unhappiness.

Help for Rape Victims

For more information on date and acquaintance rape, write:

Alternatives to Fear
1605 17th Ave.
Seattle, WA 98122

Citizens Against Crime
P.O. Box 795172
Dallas, TX 75379
Phone: (214) 390-7033

9

How to Get Down
Off the Ladder

Remember when you were a little kid and you climbed up to some high place? One of your parents told you to "Come down right now," but you didn't want to because it was fun. Or maybe you were afraid to climb down; it was harder to descend than it was to climb. Have you noticed when you are up high looking down that the distance always seems farther than when you are on the ground looking up? Once you're up there you look down, and fear begins to grip you. You feel that you can't get down. You'd like to, but you are afraid to let go of the security you have in your present position. It will mean taking risks to get back to a safer, more secure place. You are afraid to try. So you stay where you are.

Perhaps you are beginning to realize the damage and danger you face from having climbed the biological hand grenade ladder. You may desperately want to get down, but you don't think you can, or you don't know how. And, you are afraid to lose the security you feel where you are.

The First Step: New Life

The first step down the biological hand grenade ladder is to accept Jesus Christ as your Savior and Lord. Has this ever happened to you? This may be a brand new idea to you; or, you may have heard it so often it has become boring to you.

Stop for a minute and think about this. The most important decision you will ever make in life is not the selection of your life partner. It is not the choice of your occupation. The most important decision you will ever make is the decision to accept or reject Jesus Christ as your Savior. How you respond to him will determine or influence every other decision you make for the rest of your life.

I have accepted him and am not ashamed to tell you so. I was ten years old when I did it. Nobody turned the heat up in the building that night and talked about hell. Nobody promised me any rewards. I just realized that I needed Jesus Christ in my life, so I invited him in.

What I am writing here does not necessarily relate to dating. I am referring to your personal relationship with *God*.

Oh, the pain

I was splitting firewood. You know how that works. You stand an eighteen-inch log on end and drive a wedge into it with a sledge hammer. But my log kept falling over.

To solve that problem you hold the wedge with one hand while tapping it into the end of the log with the sledgehammer in the other hand. Then you step back, take a full swing with the hammer, and with one powerful blow to the wedge you drive it into the log six or eight inches, which splits the log in two.

Every time I would take my hand away from this particular log and step back to deliver the high-powered blow, the log would fall over. So I would pick the dumb thing up and do it all over again.

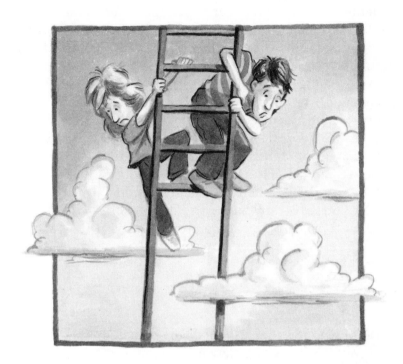

I got so tired of this I finally decided to hold the log in position with the first two fingers of my left hand, grip the sledge hammer closer to the head, and do a "one-arm job" on that log. I hit the wedge a little off center with a glancing blow, and the full impact of that ten-pound steel hammerhead came down on my fingers. I could not believe what I had done to myself.

At the hospital emergency room, I learned that I had broken one finger and almost torn the end off the other, crushing the bones in the first joint.

Our oldest daughter, Jill, was not at home when we left for the hospital. When we returned, she was shocked to see me coming in with my hand bandaged, holding it above my heart to keep it from throbbing.

I regretted going through that terrible experience. But

because I did, I had a beautiful conversation with my daughter. "Jill, I have never experienced such pain in my life," I moaned. "In the past, I have hurt my back while tobogganing and when diving. I received a painful back injury in an automobile accident. [While waiting for a light to change, my car was struck from behind by a drunken driver.] But of all the injuries I've had, none were as painful as this one.

"I realize that I have experienced only a fraction of the pain that Jesus went through to pay for my sin. Besides, mine was an accident. His was not. I did not hurt myself on purpose. Jesus suffered his pain intentionally.

"Do you have any idea why Jesus Christ voluntarily suffered a painful death on a cross? He did it for me and you. He died to pay for our sins so that we could have eternal life."

The walking dead

Do you know that if you haven't invited Jesus Christ into your life, to live inside you, you are dead?

Ephesians 2:1 says that you are "dead in trespasses and sins." Your spirit is dead and needs to be made alive. I know you don't feel dead, but that's because you don't know what it feels like to be alive, spiritually alive. To be spiritually alive means to be forgiven of all your sin and to be free from guilt. It means that you have the power of God at work in your life, because God is living in you.

You cannot do this for yourself. You can't make yourself be spiritually alive. But you can go to the person who can give you life, the Savior who died for you. He took your sin, your punishment, and your guilt.

Because he was sinless and perfect, he did not have to die for his own sin. That's why he could die in your place and pay for your sin.

You see, eternal death is the only possible payment for all your sin. But since Jesus Christ never sinned, not even once, he was able to volunteer before his Father to pay for your sin and take the death sentence for you.

But he won't take your sin unless you want him to. You have a choice. You can pay for it yourself with eternal death, or you can accept his payment by accepting him.

It will cost you something, though. It will cost you your life. He will give you his life, eternally, and he wants you to give him your life.

Complete forgiveness

How do you do this?

It is an act of faith. You believe that Jesus Christ is who he says he is, the Son of God, and that because of who he is, he took your place and died for you.

You see, the Bible says in Romans 10:9(NIV) "that if you confess with your mouth, 'Jesus is Lord' and believe in your heart that God raised him from the dead, you will be saved."

How can you possibly refuse an offer of love like that? Invite him in. He will come into you and be your Savior. You will belong to him and he will be committed to you. A very meaningful and beautiful exchange will take place: You and Christ will live for each other.

Christ offers complete and total forgiveness to you. Where else can you go to receive full pardon and forgiveness?

Would you like some more good news? This forgiveness is unconditional. That is, Jesus doesn't limit his forgiveness to only certain sins. He forgives any and all sins. So in spite of all he knows about you and all the things you've done, he will forgive you. Conversely, no matter how good you may think you are, you are not good enough to get into heaven on your own.

You can stop right now and pray. Admit to God that you are sinful and that you have broken his commandments. Ask him to forgive you, and ask Jesus Christ to come into your heart and take control of your life. This is the **first step** in getting down off the biological hand grenade ladder.

You may be thinking, *I've already done that, Bob, I am a Christian. I have accepted Jesus Christ as my Savior, but I have still gotten physically involved with my dating partner more than I should.*

Okay, so now we move to the next essential.

The Second Step: A Clear Conscience

You must have a clear conscience with God and your past, present, and future dating partners. That means you can face them without feeling guilty or ashamed.

Wow! Would that ever be terrific. Are you ready to find out how to have such beautiful freedom?

With God

First, you must have a clear conscience with God. This means that if you were to meet him face-to-face, you wouldn't feel ashamed because there were things in your life that had never been forgiven. To attain this kind of liberty you have to do two things. You must stop sinning, and you must ask God to forgive all your sins of the past.

A lot of people have taken only one of these steps. They have said, "Oh, God, I was wrong. I did this gross or immoral thing, and I want your cleansing. I admit that I did wrong."

God promises in 1 John 1:9 that "If we confess our sins, he is faithful and just to forgive us our sins, and to cleanse us from all unrighteousness."

But that's only half of clearing your conscience with God. The other part is to stop the sin. If you come to God, ask his forgiveness, and then go out and jump right back into that sin, you are making a mockery of God's forgiveness. He knows you are not sincerely sorry for your sin.

However, if you have done both of these things, you will have a clear conscience with God.

With others

Next, you must have a clear conscience with your dating partners.

If you meet persons you have dated in the past, can you look them in the eye without feeling guilty because of some of your activities with them? Or are you embarrassed about the past? When you think about a certain person, does it cause you to have lustful thoughts because of things you did together?

One man said, "Every time I go to my best friend's house, I have lustful thoughts about his wife. Before she married him, she dated me, and we got sexually involved. Now every time I see her that's all I can think about. It's difficult to be around her, because I keep trying to restart the old fire in her, but she won't respond. I even find myself hoping that she and her husband will have marriage problems so she will confide in me. That way I might get close to her. I know these thoughts are wrong. I feel guilty about them, but I can't seem to overcome them."

To get rid of guilt and overcome lustful thoughts, you need a supernatural source of power. Jesus Christ is that source of power. He can make changes inside you that will completely rearrange and revolutionize you. But just accepting him and asking God's forgiveness is not all there is to it.

If you have gone up the biological hand grenade ladder with one or more people in the past, you have the responsibility of contacting each of them. You must admit you were wrong and ask their forgiveness.

Jesus refers to this principle in Matthew 5:23 (NIV): "Therefore, if you are offering your gift at the altar and there remember that your brother has something against you, leave your gift there in front of the altar. First go and be reconciled to your brother; then come and offer your gift."

God is not interested in my religious activities or financial gifts if I have offended a brother and not made things right with him. And how do I make things right? By asking the offended person to forgive my offense and by repaying any damages where possible.

To be able to look every person in the eye without guilt, you must have a clear conscience toward them as well as toward God. And the Lord wants us to strive to live with a clear conscience.

Look at Acts 24:16: "And herein do I exercise myself, to have always a conscience void of offense toward God, and toward men." Another translation says: "I strive always to keep my conscience clear before God and man" (NIV). Notice it does not stop with just God; the verse includes "and toward man."

The apostle Paul is emphasizing the importance of having total freedom of conscience, which is possible only when there is nothing between you and God or you and another person.

One guy asked, "Do I really have to go back to that person? If I have asked God's forgiveness, isn't that enough?"

Suppose a good friend comes to your house to visit. There's a fifty-dollar bill lying on your dresser, which you have been saving for something special. After your friend is gone, you can't find your money. You don't even suspect that he may have taken it, because he is not only your friend, he is also a leader in your church group. So you assume that you must have misplaced the money.

Later, you learn from someone else that your friend did, in fact, take the money. Since you can't prove he took it, you don't say anything to him. You pray for him, asking God to make him feel guilty for his wrong.

One Sunday your pastor preaches on the Ten Commandments and comes down super hard on stealing. After church, you overhear you thieving friend telling someone how the pastor's sermon really hit home with him, and that he asked God to forgive him for all of his sin. Now he is feeling much better.

How would you feel about this guy the next time he was leading a church activity? You would think he was a phony.

But suppose he had come to you and said, "Hey, man, I did something I'm really ashamed of. I took fifty bucks from you. I sure am sorry. Here's your money. Will you forgive me for stealing it?"

Ah, now that's a different story. If he had done this and then led a church activity, you would probably think, *Now there's a real Christian. He lives it.*

You see, God's way to really be free from guilt is for us to clear it up with the person we have wronged as well as with God. When we sin against God, we must ask his forgiveness. When we wrong others, we must ask their forgiveness also.

Asking forgiveness

I have a practical suggestion for asking forgiveness. Don't put it in writing. Don't write a letter to a previous dating partner asking her to forgive you for your sinful activities with her. Others may read it.

Don't even go see her face-to-face. I have known people who have gone to a former dating partner intending to ask forgiveness for "going up the ladder" while they were dating. Their intention was to do something spiritual and scriptural, but Satan took advantage of the renewed contact and lured them right back into the same sin.

Use the telephone.

Before you call your former partner, think through what you are going to say. Don't go into detail about past activities. All you have to do is admit that you were wrong in not being the kind of person you should have been while you were dating. Admit that you did not treat her the way God wanted you to. Then ask, "Will you forgive me?"

Notice I did not suggest that you say "I'm sorry," or "I

hope you'll forgive me." You should say, "I was wrong and I want to know, will you forgive me?" This is a question. It requests an answer.

If the other person says, "Yes, I forgive you," whew! This is when the freedom comes.

You may be asking, "What if she won't forgive me?"

Now, there's a vital question, and here's the answer: "Would you be willing to let me know when you do forgive me?"

You have now taken the responsibility off your shoulders and placed it on hers. You have done what God requires you to do. It is now the responsibility of the other person to respond the way God wants her to respond.

What if she says, "There's nothing to forgive. I enjoyed it. We were in love and it was right for us at the time. We parted friends."

You might say, "I enjoyed it too, at the time. But since that time I have realized that it grieved the Lord. I was wrong to have used you for my own pleasure. I was thinking only of myself and not of you. Will you forgive me for taking unfair advantage of you?"

I believe there is one other person you should tell about the major events in your past: your potential marriage partner. For example, if you have had an abortion, you should tell your dating partner if the relationship is moving toward marriage. Why? Because your major life experiences will affect your mutual trust, the depth of your communication, and ultimately your spiritual intimacy.

At a family camp in Wisconsin, a lady said to me, "It's really true, Bob. Potential mates must be honest about their past to the person they plan to marry, or it could destroy the relationship.

"My nephew married a woman whom he thought was a virgin. A year later he found out she had previously had a child, and he later divorced her."

If your dating partner is going to hold your past against you, you certainly want to know it before you are married. Your dating partner needs the opportunity to forgive you, and at the very least needs protection from the terrible shock of learning about your past from someone else.

Basic to all of this is the fact that a loving relationship is built on trust, and trust is established and nourished by openness and honesty.

10

Give Yourself Away

If you have previously climbed the biological hand grenade ladder but are now making every effort to get down, and if you have taken the first two steps explained in the previous chapter, you have made some major progress. But, there is one further step you must take. That third step is to apply Romans 12:1, 2 to your life:

> I beseech you therefore, brethren, by the mercies of God, that you present your bodies a living sacrifice, holy, acceptable to God, which is your reasonable service. Do not be conformed to this world, but be transformed by the renewing of your mind, that you may prove what is that good and acceptable and perfect will of God.

You may have heard these two verses so many times you could almost quote them sideways, but let's look closely at them, particularly at four key words.

The First Key: Body

Our first key word from this text is *body*. Your body was created and given to you by God, and he wants you to give it back to him. He created every living cell in your body. He lovingly designed every intricate part, and he wants you to dedicate each part—your entire body—to him.

Be specific

Now, I'm a guy who doesn't like to take things for granted. I try not to assume anything, and I always endeavor to be very specific. Since God is always precise in what he says and does, I think God wants you to be specific in dedicating your body to him.

Begin at the top of your head and start working your way down. You won't drop down far until you hit something that needs to be dedicated—your eyes.

> O Father, here are my eyes. I dedicate these eyes to you. Now that they are consecrated to you, I pray that I will look only at things that will build me up and not at things that will draw me away from you, things I shouldn't look at or read. Please help me to watch only things on TV that will strengthen my character and my relationship with you rather than things that will plant immoral thoughts or encourage wrong behavior. I dedicate my eyes to you.

Have you ever dedicated your eyes to God? If some guys did this, they would have to throw away all of the literature they have stashed under their mattress at home.

Here is a meaningful verse from Psalm 101:3: "I will set nothing wicked before mine eyes."

How about Job 31:1 (NIV)? "I made a covenant with my eyes; not to look lustfully at a girl."

> Here are my lips, Father. I pray that I will say only things that will be encouraging and comforting to others, things that will lift them up or exhort them to draw close to you. Help me not to talk about sex or tell dirty jokes and to keep my tongue in my own mouth.

Here are my hands, Lord. I dedicate them to you. I pray that they will be used to do positive and constructive things for you by helping others. Please help me to keep them from doing anything they shouldn't do or touching anything they should not touch.

As I said before, a guy's hands are "wired." His hands are part of his sexual equipment. He loves to touch a girl in those sensitive places. He likes to feel the texture of certain areas of her body. Just the touching can arouse a major hunger in him.

Friend, have you dedicated your hands to God?

If you are a girl: "Father, here are those sensitive spots around my neck and ear lobes."

That's part of your sexual equipment, right? The word floats around, you know: "All you have to do is nibble on her ear and she 'goes bananas.'" Have you ever dedicated that part of your body to God?

Women: "Father, here are my sex organs."

Men: "Here are my sex organs, Lord. They belong to you and I will use them only to bring glory to you. You created them exlusively for marriage, so I will save them for that special relationship."

"Here are my feet, Lord. I dedicate them to you so that they won't go anywhere they should not go."

Dedicated head to toe; that's what God wants.

A date with her father

Here is the scene. Henrietta has been invited to go out with Herman. Then Herman gets the startling news; he has to ask her father's permission to take her out!

He says, "I don't want to go out with your dad; I want to go out with you."

But Herman calls her father and makes an appointment to see him. When they get together, her father asks him some important questions.

Henrietta's dad wants to know a little about this guy's background. He wants to get an indication of his basic attitudes and intentions, to get a reading of his "spiritual temperature." He doesn't want his daughter going out with someone who has concupiscence. Now obviously, the dad can't say to him, "Do you have a strong desire for sex?" But the dad may be able to discern if this guy has a hunger in his heart for the Lord.

If her dad says, "Yes, our daughter may go out with you," how then should Herman approach this girl and their date, if he has dedicated his body to God? Something like the following should happen, I think, to plant the roots of a right relationship.

Start out right

As they approach his car, he will open the door for her.
Wow! Some guy!
Well, God says in 1 Corinthians 13 that love has good manners.
After he is in the car but before he starts the engine, he says, "Henrietta, I want you to know I told your dad about the most important decision I have ever made in my whole life: to accept Jesus Christ as my Savior. But before we go on this date, I want to tell you something. I have dedicated my life and my body to God. I promised God that I would reserve myself 100 percent for my life partner, and that I would not do anything with a girl that would displease the Lord. I'm committed to wait until I have vowed my vows. Henrietta, will you help me keep my promise to God tonight on this date?"
Wouldn't that be something?
You say, "Yeah, that's really something."
If the girl is also a sincere Christian, she will say, "You can count on me, Herman. I have made that same commitment in my life. I'd like you to help me keep my promise, too."
"It's a deal," Herman responds.

The Second Key: Beseech

Let's look at Romans 12:1 again: "I beseech you therefore, brethren, by the mercies of God . . . " Stop at the word *beseech*. What in the world does that mean? This is not your ordinary twentieth-century word. You probably don't hear any of your friends using it. "Oh, Mom, please, I beseech you to let me go out tonight!"

Beseech means "beg."

Do you know who wrote the Book of Romans in the Bible? God had the apostle Paul write it. We are not talking about some guy who just got his name mentioned in the Bible. This is the man who wrote over a dozen books of the Bible.

Suppose you are home alone one afternoon after school. There's a knock on your front door. You open it and find the apostle Paul standing there dressed as he was when he lived on the earth. He doesn't look "tuned in." He doesn't have on any T-shirt with lettering. But you know it's he, so you invite him in.

You lead the way into the living room, offer him a seat, and you sit down in your favorite chair. But he doesn't sit down. Instead, he walks over to you, gets down on his knees, looks you square in the eye, and begs you to do something. This godly man begs you to dedicate your body to God as a "living sacrifice."

As you look at him, you can see the compassion and concern on his face. He really cares. He does not want you to be a sexual sacrifice. He wants you to be a living sacrifice for Jesus Christ. He wants you to be a dynamic example of what Jesus Christ can do in the life of a person like you.

The Third Key: Mind

Now let's check out another key word from Romans 12:2: "Do not be conformed to this world, but be transformed by the renewing of your mind."

Did you catch it? The word is *mind*.

Your body is not actually what gives you trouble. It's your mind that starts it all. Proverbs 23:7 says that "as a man thinks in his heart, so is he." Of course, you don't think with your heart muscle. When Solomon uses the word *heart* here he is talking about what you think in your innermost thoughts.

Paul then comes along and says you need to have your mind renewed. Why? Because it is full of corruption, selfishness, greed, and lust.

We have heard a lot about brainwashing in recent years. Some political and military leaders in foreign countries use brainwashing techniques to win followers.

Brainwashing involves saturating people's minds with the philosophy or ideas that you want them to accept. Under certain circumstances, you can gain complete control of another person with this technique.

I believe many teenagers have been brainwashed by the philosophy of the world around them through television, movies, music, magazines, and friends. Consequently, they need to have their brains "washed" by the Lord to be freed from mind control by the world and Satan.

Jesus said that murder and adultery begin in our thoughts and attitudes. This is why we need to be washed or renewed in our minds.

How do we achieve that? Look at this: "Thy word have I hid in my heart, that I might not sin against thee" (Ps. 119:11). "Now you are clean through the word which I have spoken to you" (John 15:3).

You "take a bath" in the word of God. In other words, you saturate yourself with it, read it, study it, memorize it. It has to become part of your very life.

What I am describing here is to become so saturated with the truth and wisdom of God that it is automatically helping to guide your thoughts, reactions, attitudes, and decisions. You have laced it into your subconscious mind, your "heart."

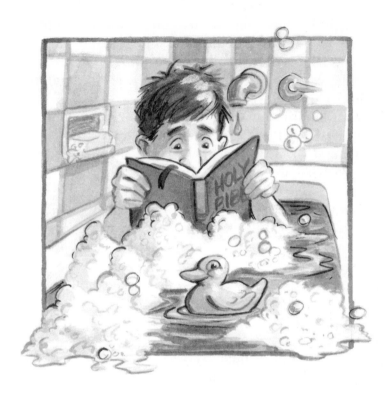

Here are some suggestions for what to start memorizing: 2 Corinthians 10:3–6, Ephesians 6:10–13, Psalm 119:9 and 11. Then, if you are really serious about hiding God's word in your heart, memorize Romans 6 and 7. Yes, the entire chapters. They are dynamite!

Have you noticed how music can control your feelings? Music can make you feel sad or happy, tense or calm, peppy or relaxed. Do you know what else it can do? It can help renew your mind.

"Oh, oh, Bob, there you go, getting off on that kick," some teenagers will say. "Just leave my music alone, okay?"

Although extensive studies have been done on the effects of music, I won't take time here to discuss them in detail. At this point, I just want you to look at Ephesians

5:19 where God encourages "speaking to one another in psalms and hymns and spiritual songs, singing and making melody in your heart to the Lord."

Notice the writer mentions two things: psalms, which are the word of God, and hymns and spiritual songs —God's word and spiritual music.

What kind of music do you listen to? This will help to determine whether or not the garbage is driven out of your mind. If you listen to the kind of music that promotes sexual freedom, anti-authority, drug use, and do whatever feels good to you, you will not come down off the ladder.

Your brain is one of God's most marvelous creations. Judith Hooper and Dick Teresi, in their book *The Three Pound Universe* (New York: Macmillan, 1986, p. 36, 37), say that the average brain weighs three and one-half pounds. It has up to one hundred billion cells and one hundred trillion synaptic connections. You can hold it in the palm of your hand; but a computer with the same number of bytes of memory would be a hundred stories tall and would cover the state of Texas.

Your brain can store one hundred billion facts, except during exams. And it is Satan's focal point. Satan loves to fill your mind with impure thoughts and crowd out godly ideas. When you give in to lustful reflection, it will cause you to forget other things and make you inconsistent. James 1:8 says that "a double minded man is unstable in all his ways."

That's why Ephesians 4:23 says: "be renewed in the spirit of your mind." God wants you to think as Christ thought when he was on the earth. "Let this mind be in you, which was also in Christ Jesus" (Phil. 2:5). He didn't lust. He didn't harbor jealousy or resentment. God wants you to be like him. So if you put more and more of his book into your mind, you're going to start thinking as he thinks. Wouldn't that be beautiful?

The Fourth Key: Will of God

Look again at Romans 12:2. We haven't finished the verse yet. There is one more key we want to look at. "And do not be conformed to this world, but be transformed by the renewing of your mind, that you may prove what the *will of God* is, that which is good and acceptable and perfect" (NAS).

What is the will of God? That we should live in obedience to his word by doing what is good and acceptable and perfect.

God wants you to do his will instead of your will. He wants you to surrender your will to him. Give up what you want to do and do what he wants. Our natural tendency is to carry out our own will, go our own way. But God wants us to give our will to him through a voluntary act of surrender. Do you have a surrendered will or are you still living your life according to your own will?

When I was in high school, although I was a Christian, I had not surrendered my will to God and determined to live my life totally for him. As I grew in my understanding of God through the study of his word, I began to see that I could place my trust in him and find the security I wanted and needed. He could be trusted when no one else could because he loved me unconditionally and would only do what was best for me as his child. But I was still unwilling to surrender my will to him.

Most of us resist giving in to God's will. It's our pride that keeps us from giving ourselves totally to God. "God opposes the proud but gives grace to the humble" (James 4:6). Do you want God to oppose you? I don't. "The sacrifices of God are a broken spirit: a broken and a contrite heart, O God, thou wilt not despise" (Ps. 51:17). And, "The LORD is nigh [near] unto them that are of a broken heart; and saveth such as be of a contrite spirit"(Ps. 34:18).

The word *heart* in the Bible is widely used to mean the

will, the feelings, and the intellect. God wants us to set aside our pride and the determination to do what we want to do, and do what he wants instead.

When we have done this, he becomes our Lord (boss) as well as our Savior. Our top priority is no longer what we want but rather what he wants. We now want to obey his word and love him in return.

But we can't prove our love to God apart from obedience. Jesus said, "If you love me, keep my commandments" (John 14:15). "He who has my commandments and keeps them, it is he who loves me" (John 14:21 NKJV).

Traps to Avoid

Christian young people will face some seemingly innocent choices, but they must make crucial decisions not to become involved in these "harmless" activities. Look out for some subtle traps, and avoid them.

"Traps! What traps?" you might ask?

Falling for a non-Christian

One "biggie" in which many Christians get caught is that of falling for a person who is not a Christian.

"Oh, good night, here we go again. All you Christian leaders jump on this one and beat it to death."

That's right, because God is so smart he knows it won't work. If you are a Christian and date and marry a non-Christian, you will wind up being miserable. Your spirit doesn't match with the other person's spirit. You are heading in two different directions. Your goals and priorities are not the same. You will never experience the depth of oneness that God wants you to experience if you and your mate are going in different directions.

If your allegiance is toward God and you are married to someone who is living for himself or herself, someone who is "turned off" to God, you can't have oneness with that person. This is why the Bible says: "Do not be unequally yoked together with unbelievers" (2 Cor. 6:14).

This would be like an ox and a donkey harnessed together. They cannot work together. They don't walk the same pace or pull with the same power. A donkey can be stubborn, while an ox is a patient animal. They will just battle each other or go 'round and 'round in circles.

I'm so glad I have a Christian wife; we have oneness. When you have the kind of togetherness my wife and I enjoy, it's hard to know where one person ends and the other begins. There's one pulse-beat, the ultimate joy of marriage.

A negative background

Another trap in which you could get caught is to become tied to a partner with a dysfunctional home life. This is especially dangerous for a girl. If you date a guy with an unstable background and an unhappy past, you may be tempted to fall into a very subtle trap.

God has given you a mother instinct. You have a natural desire to take care of someone who feels rejected or who has trouble keeping his life straight. You will have a tendency to feel sorry for a guy like this. Thinking he needs you to take care of him will make you feel good about yourself. He may even tell you that he needs you and that he can't survive without you.

You will think, *Oh, you poor guy. Nobody cares about you. Nobody loves you or accepts you. I'll accept you. I'll take care of you.* You envision that he's going to go "eat some worms" if you don't show him how much you care.

Meanwhile, he's thinking, *All right! I'll accept you, too, "baby." Come here.*

I like to imagine that each of us has a cup down inside our heart. Each person's cup is filled with either love or selfishness. The cup of a person raised in an unloving or unhappy environment is likely filled with selfishness, resentment, and anger. If such a man doesn't have love in the "cup" inside him, what will eventually come out of him? When he needs to respond with love he won't be able to. If there is rebellion, bitterness, resentment, or self-ishness inside, that's what will come out.

The Tragedy of Rejection

I was meeting with a group of about seventy teenagers in an open discussion when one guy suddenly began to cry. Now, you have to be going through something awfully heavy to burst into tears right in front of every-one. The others just sat and stared at the floor for a few moments. After a brief pause, the discussion continued. When the meeting was over, I gave the guy a ride home, along with several other kids.

When he got out of my car, I stepped out and asked if he needed to talk.

He replied, "No, I can't tell you."

"If you ever need me, you know how to get in touch with me," I said.

The next morning the guy called me and said, "Bob, the thing I wouldn't tell you last night is that I was over at my girlfriend's house recently. After her parents left, she came indecently exposed into the room where I was waiting. I immediately went out the front door as fast as I could go."

"You mean you are a teenage guy with red blood in your veins," I marveled, "and you ran out the front door? Man, I can't believe this!"

He said that as he headed down the street, the girl came to the door and yelled loudly enough to be heard three or four houses down the block, "Nobody cares!"

That poor girl, who was looking for love and affection through a sexual experience, "hollered her heart out" that night. She expressed the pain and anguish she was feeling deep inside. She was hoping to find something to permeate the emptiness in her heart. She was willing to settle for a hollow substitute that could never satisfy her longing. This is exactly what the world urges us to do.

The teenage guy did the right thing. If he had given in to her advances, it would have made things worse for both of them. He would have added guilt and disappointment to her frustration. Of course, he, too, would face the consequence of guilt. But he stood up like a real man and refused to give in to temptation.

That situation reminds me of a young man named Joseph whose story is told in the Book of Genesis. Joseph was a servant in the house of Potiphar. Day after day Potiphar's wife begged Joseph to go to bed with her. But he refused. His life was totally dedicated to God.

One day the two of them were alone in the house. She called Joseph into her bedroom (remember, he was a servant). When he walked in, she grabbed his shirt and pleaded with him to go to bed with her. She hung on so tightly that he had to slip out of his shirt to get away.

Talk about commitment! That man went through all kinds of pain and turmoil, including several years in prison, because he refused to give in to temptation. He lived an exemplary life before all the people in the Egyptian home, and God later honored him with the position of prime minister of Egypt.

God recorded these events in the life of Joseph as an example to us. He wants us to realize that we, too, can live this kind of exemplary life. But we are not left to live it by ourselves. If you have the supernatural source of power in you that comes with being a Christian, you are equipped to resist temptation. You can turn to God for help. He will give you the inner courage and fortitude to say no to sin. He will make it possible for you to live the way he wants you to live. But you've gotta ask.

When the guy who had burst into tears called me that morning, he told me the rest of the story. His girlfriend's mother had called to let him know that after he left their house, her daughter had swallowed a whole bottle of sleeping pills. When she went to wake her daughter for school, this poor mother found her daughter dead.

That brokenhearted girl felt so rejected and unloved by everyone around her that she gave up all hope of a meaningful life.

A Fresh Start

Do you need life? Do you need forgiveness? Would you like a brand new start with a clean slate?

"Oh, but you don't know what I have done," you may respond. "I have been immoral or had an abortion or participated in activities that are too shameful to even mention."

That's exactly why Jesus Christ died. He paid for all sin. That's the reason you can turn to him right now. You can call on him right where you are. He will respond to you so quickly that it will leave you flabbergasted.

If you understand that you are incomplete without him and that you do need forgiveness, stop reading, put this book down, bow before him in prayer, and ask him to forgive you and to be your Savior.

If you are not sure how to pray or what to say, remember it is not your prayer that saves you or cleanses you from sin; Jesus Christ forgives and cleanses from sin. But if you need some guidance, pray something like this:

Father, I realize that I need your Son, Jesus Christ. I'm a sinner in need of forgiveness. I admit it. Please forgive all my sin. Right now, I bow in your presence and invite Jesus Christ to be my Savior and my Lord.

Thank you, Father, for cleansing me from sin. Thank you for sending your Son to be my Lord and Savior. I want you to be in complete control of my life.

I pray this in Jesus' name. Amen.

If you prayed a prayer similar to this one and you meant it with all your heart, you have been forgiven.

How do I know? Because the Bible says: "If you confess with your mouth the Lord Jesus and believe in your heart that God has raised him from the dead, you will be saved. For whoever calls upon the name of the Lord shall be saved" (Rom. 10:9, 13).

You have just taken the most important step in getting down off the ladder. Now God will give you the power to take the other steps.

11

How to Know When It's Love

Once a person understands the concept of the biological hand grenade ladder and is aware of some of the pitfalls that may be encountered in that kind of relationship, the natural question that follows is, How do you know when it's real love?

There are no simple answers to this question, but there are some indicators that will help to determine the difference between genuine love and a counterfeit.

Do you like poetry? I do. Here's one I thought might really hit a tender spot in your heart:

> At sweet sixteen I first began
> To ask the good Lord for a man.
> At seventeen, I recall,
> I wanted someone strong and tall.
> The Christmas I reached eighteen,
> I fancied someone tall and lean.
> And then at nineteen I was sure
> I'd fall for someone more mature.
> At twenty I thought I'd find
> Romance with someone with a "mind."
> I retrogressed at twenty-one,
> And found college boys most fun.
> My viewpoint changed at twenty-two,

> When "one man only" was my cue.
> I broke my heart at twenty-three,
> And asked for someone kind to me.
> Then begged at blasé twenty-four
> For anyone who would not bore.
> Now, Lord, I'm twenty-five;
> Just send me someone who's alive.

Often people do things out of desperation. The writer of this poem seems to have become reckless. She sounds willing to accept anything that walks and talks with a deep voice. She might be willing to do almost anything to get a man, especially someone to whom she is attracted.

Naturally, if you care about someone of the opposite sex, you want to do everything just right. You want to make a good impression so that person will be attracted to you. You try to look right, act right, and smell right. But just making a good impression and being greatly impressed yourself does not mean that there is any love between the two of you.

In fact, many teenagers have been deceived into thinking they are in love with someone when actually they are just attracted to the other person's surface personality. This is what we call infatuation. Often, when they *really get to know* that other person, they realize that they are not in love after all.

There are three T's by which I like to measure any relationship that help reveal its depth. Each T represents a test by which love may be appraised: treatment, time, and trust.

There are actually more indicators of genuine love, but these three are usually very easy to spot. If you watch for them, they may help you avoid getting trapped in a wrong relationship.

Treatment

The first test is the test of treatment. The way you treat someone reveals, more than anything, how you really feel about that person. There are several areas included in how you treat someone you are dating.

Verbal treatment

How do you talk to each other? Haven't you heard two kids who are dating just tear into each other? She'll pick at him for a while, and he will respond with, "Oh, yeah, woman?" Then he cuts her down. She gets angry and lashes back at him. They begin to turn up the volume. The louder they get, the more sarcastic they become.

Some people use humor to say things that they wouldn't dare say seriously. When the other person takes offense, they usually reply with a defensive comment such as, "Aw, be a sport. I was just joking."

A group of us were meeting in a restaurant. Everyone was seated, but we were waiting for one guy's girlfriend. She had been gaining a few pounds here and there, and he had tried to encourage her to lose them. When she came through the door, he called out to her, "Over here, honey. Pull up a couple of chairs and sit down."

She looked hurt and offended. He said, "What's the matter, sweetie, can't you take a joke?"

I knew a guy who had a serious case of acne. It didn't matter to his girlfriend. She was really attracted to his personality and never made a disparaging remark about him. However, he sometimes belittled her with humor. She took it for a while, but one day stopped him cold when she said, "You've got so many pockmarks I've decided to call you moonface."

Outside the door of a college class I was teaching, I overheard a couple talking one day. I took special note of the tone of the conversation. A few days later when the girl came in for counseling, I asked, "Are you in love?"

Her eyes brightened as she said, "Wow, am I ever!"

"Well, I'm not the Holy Spirit nor even a prophet," I remarked, "but I would like to challenge your response."

"On what basis?" she asked.

"I heard the two of you talking in the hall the other day. Oh, boy, were you sarcastic with each other. I don't believe that two people who sincerely love one another will attack each other like that," I explained.

I am not saying you can't have fun. I love to laugh and I love to make people laugh, but not at the expense of others by publicly embarrassing or belittling them. Verbal treatment is an indicator of the true feelings and attitudes of love and respect.

Physical treatment

Another thing to consider in the area of treatment is the way two people treat each other physically. Is the guy running for the award of "Grand Octopus of the Twentieth Century," or "Mr. Hands of America?" Such a guy usually uses the line, "If you love me, you'll prove it."

That line is as old as your great-grandma. But one day it suddenly hit me that it is a true statement, not the way guys usually mean it, but true nevertheless. If you sincerely love someone, your attitudes and actions will prove it. Jesus even made such a statement: "If you love me, keep my commandments" (John 14:15).

Are you in a dating relationship right now? If you are, is it centered mainly around a physical relationship? Where do you spend most of your time? What do you do when you are alone?

When I talk like this, some guys get mad at me. One six-foot, four-inch high school guy in Texas walked up to me after a meeting where I had explained some of these principles. He said, "Hey, man, what are you trying to do, turn all of our women into 'Frigidaires'?"

Don't get me wrong. Sure, I'm "old" and married and ordained, and it probably seems to you that I'm out of touch with reality. But I am trying to help you see that there is a trap waiting for you out there. Most teenagers are blind to the hooks that are lurking behind some very attractive bait.

"Oh, that bait looks tempting! It smells good. It looks good. It feels good to touch. It seems so harmless and so inviting. How could it possibly be destructive?"

The most deceptive thing of all is that the closer you get, the better it looks. The trouble is that you don't find out it is attached to a trap until you've been caught and it is too late. One day you look around and can't figure out why in the world your life is in such shambles. Where did I go wrong, you wonder?

I have had opportunity to speak in both public and Christian high schools, colleges, and universities, and I have repeatedly watched the response of the students change from skepticism to agreement as I explain these concepts.

At the start, when I talk about these things, the students think, "Oh, brother, this guy is a real weirdo." Gradually, as they listen, some will begin to nod in agreement. They have experienced the things I am talking about. Eventually, tears begin to trickle down the faces of many.

You may want to "live it up" now, but if you do, it will take years to "live it down." During my entire years of ministry I have never met one married person who has said, "I wish I had 'lived it up' when I was dating. I wish I had been more sexually active." But I could fill several large auditoriums with people who have said, "Oh, how I regret my past."

Eliminate the physical part of your relationship, and see how your dating partner responds. See if he or she starts to get irritable and touchy and says to you, "Our relationship is not based on physical involvement. I can take it or leave it." But stop the physical activities and see what happens. There may be some arm-biting and maybe you should check a backyard to see if all the bark is gone off the trees.

Emotional treatment

If your relationship is actually built on love, it will include good manners and will involve doing kind and creative things for that other person. It will be built on unselfishness.

I love to tell this story. I know a couple in their seventies who live in Ohio. They have the smallest kitchen table I've ever seen. If three people are invited for dinner, they almost have to eat in shifts.

While spending a weekend in their home, I was in the bathroom shaving when they called me to breakfast. In the kitchen were three places set at this tiny table. I thought, *Wow, here we go.* When we sat down, all of our knees touched.

The man said, "Let's ask the blessing on the food."

I closed my eyes, and then I heard a little noise during the prayer.

Now, when I went to a Christian college, I was taught that if you peek during prayer, you will go blind. So I thought, *Well, I'll risk one eye.*

When I looked up, I saw his hand coming around the sugar bowl, her hand coming around the cereal box, and they grasped hands.

When he finished praying, they both stood up. Now, remember how close we were. They leaned toward each other, almost got me in the process, kissed each other right there in front of me, and then sat back down.

When it was time to leave for church, because it was winter, he went out and moved the car from the garage to the side of the house. He left the heater on to make the car nice and "toasty" for his wife. He came back in the house, helped her with her coat, helped her out to the car, opened the door for her, and helped her into the car. When we arrived at the church, he opened the car door, helped her out, and then opened the door of the church for her.

She said, "Thanks, Love," and then waited just inside the church door while he parked the car—waiting for him to help her with her coat.

Do you know what went on inside me as I watched all

this? "Oh, Lord, that's the kind of relationship I want to have with Ruth when we are in our seventies."

Lovers will treat one another like that.

Time

The next T in the test of love is time.

I was standing near another man in an auto parts store when a beautiful young woman walked by. As she passed him he said "O-o-o-h! I'm in love!"

But was he? Not on your life. He may have been "in lust" for a moment there, but he certainly was not in love.

How do you feel about love at first sight? You may say you believe in it, because you know someone who married on impulse, and it lasted. They saw each other and said, "There's the one. Oh, Lord, thank you. Yup, that's the person I'm supposed to marry. Thank you, God, for answered prayer." They got married and they are still married to each other. But I can guarantee that this is a rare exception.

Do you know why I don't believe in love at first sight? Because love is not a feeling. Love is an act of the will. Infatuation is a feeling. Love is a growing relationship that requires time to develop.

Love is action. God says love is long-suffering and kind. It is the way you treat another person. Feelings are temporary. Feelings rise and fall with moods and circumstances. Love is a choice. You choose to treat someone with kindness and consideration.

Oh, I'm not saying that genuine love has no feelings. It does have feelings, fantastic feelings. When you are deeply in love with someone, you will feel some feelings you never felt before. But if this love is real, those feelings are controlled. Sincere love will never intentionally hurt the one being loved, unless it is in that person's best interest. Unfeigned love always thinks of the other person's welfare.

On what are you basing your choices? Are you making your choices on what you see at a glance? It takes time to get to know someone, longer to love.

Bulldozers and race cars

Did you ever watch a bulldozer at work? It never moves fast. Listen to that great big diesel engine "hum" with a steady drone as the huge, iron creature moves slowly forward, pushing down large trees as if they were toothpicks.

Compare that massive bulldozer with a high-powered racing car or a dragster. Unlike the dozer, the dragster does not have a steady droning sound. It's more of a vrrroom, vrrroom, vrrroom!!! When all of that power is unleashed into the rear wheels, you hear the deafening roar of the engine and the screeching, squalling, screaming sound of rubber against blacktop as the rear end of that high-tech machine fishtails from side to side down an asphalt strip.

I have a buddy named Dave who has taken first in his class in a national drag race. After one race Dave told me, "Bob, we spent hundreds of hours and thousands of dollars getting the engine in that car built and tuned to perfection. We rolled that baby out on the strip, waited for the lights on the 'Christmas tree' to change colors, popped the clutch . . . and blew the engine."

I've seen a lot of relationships like that. They start out fast and furious, go too far, too fast, and "blow up" not very far down the road.

One day while looking out the window of my office at the college, I saw a group of sixty to seventy students in a circle. I thought, *Oh no, there's a fight. This is a Christian school, and there's a fight in the parking lot.* So I hustled downstairs, out the front door, and worked my way through the crowd to get to the center. As I was looking for the battered bodies of the people who were "whaling the tar" out of one another, all I saw was a small woman standing there holding out her left hand so the sunlight would sparkle off that little "rock" which had been placed on her finger.

Now you may think, *Awww, what a tender little story.* But you don't know the details. Number one, the engaged couple were from opposite ends of the country. Number two, this was the third week of September, and they had never met before coming to school that semester. Here they were, already in love. He had already popped the question, she had already accepted, and he had already taken her to the jewelry store. They were engaged.

The great deception

Girls, did you know that some guys will use an engagement ring to "put the moves" on you?

A girl instinctively has a built-in sense of reserve. She has a sensitive conscience and a natural tendency to hold back from giving herself to a physical relationship with a guy, unless there is some kind of commitment between them.

I have talked with dozens of girls who have been given a diamond, and as a result have given in to sex, thinking they were giving themselves to their future husbands. Later the engagements were broken, and they walked away feeling cheated and "used." (Remember chapter 2 where we discussed defrauding.)

Once you become engaged, there is a tendency to drop the barriers, thinking that this is the person you are going to marry. But remember two things. First, engagement is a time to get to know each other in depth, spiritually and intellectually. Second, God says clearly that the sexual relationship is for marriage, not engagement.

This happens occasionally. My phone rings, and the voice on the other end says, "Hey, watcha doin' Friday night?"

I may be crazy but I'm not stupid, so I respond with, "What did you have in mind?"

They say, "Well, we'd like to get married this Friday

night. Would you be willing to do it?" (There's nothing like planning ahead, right?)

Here is one that beats all, though. I answered the phone, and a lady said, "I found your church in the yellow pages. Are you busy tonight?"

I asked her my standard question, "Well, what did you have in mind?"

"We want to get married and wondered if you would perform the ceremony."

"Oh, dear lady, you probably have no idea what it takes to get married in this church," I said. "We really put you through it. You have to meet with the pastor, who checks out your 'spiritual temperature.' Then he really punishes you and sends you to see me. You have to meet with me for four, one-hour sessions. I have several questionnaires you must fill out and which include about seventy-five questions.

"You must also listen to several cassette tapes regarding marriage, which I then discuss with you and your fiancé, in depth.

"Because we believe that marriage is the second-most important decision people make in their whole lives, we want to be sure you are not rushing into it totally unprepared."

Hey, are you in a hurry? God isn't. I would like to challenge you to be like a bulldozer instead of the vrrroom, vrrroom, vrrroom! This is the one, Lord. Thank you. Drop this machine into first gear. Whew, boy, I've gotta get me a man. I'm a senior. There's one, and he looks like he's got money.

Some guys get so desperate to find a wife they begin to think, "I don't care if she has one leg, I'll take her." And some fellas conclude God has forgotten them or isn't interested in their dating life and whether or not they find a wife. Some young men may even have the mistaken idea that God doesn't want them to have an attractive wife. They fear that because the Bible says all who live godly will suffer, maybe that means if they turn their dating life over to the Lord, he might give them someone really ugly, and say, "Okay, if you love me, marry that."

God is not at all like that. In fact, he is just the opposite. Look at Psalm 37:4: "Delight thyself also in the Lord; and he shall give thee the desires of thine heart."

God knows the deepest desires of your heart. He also knows where those desires can lead you. He wants you to respond to the desires that will result in the greatest joy in your life. He wants to spare you the painful results of following the wrong desires.

If you rush into a relationship, you won't give the Lord time to show you whether or not this is the right relationship for you. He wants you to know that person intellectually, emotionally, and spiritually, If you don't, you are liable to have a rude awakening later.

I am convinced that time is one of the test tracks God has established to reveal whether or not something or someone is really for you.

She walked into my office and said, "Oh, Bob, I finally met one. This guy is so spiritual that he prays on our dates. In fact, through taking your class, we have realized it's true; a lot of couples can pray at the beginning of a date but not at the end because of what they have done on the date. We pray at the end of our dates. We also read the chapter of Proverbs that corresponds to the day of the month. If we go out on the seventeenth, we read the seventeenth chapter. And, we memorize Scripture together. Wow! Thank you, Lord!"

About a month later, he popped the big question. She accepted and joined the girl in the parking lot whom I mentioned a few pages back. Everybody gathered around to offer their congratulations.

During Christmas vacation he went home with her to be "checked out" by her mom and dad. One evening while her parents were away, he snuggled up to her on the couch and whispered in her ear, "Could we start our honeymoon tonight?"

After the Christmas break, a knock came on my office

door. There stood this twenty-three-year-old woman. With tears streaming down her face, she said, "Bob, I remember your little statement; 'Time is one of the greatest test tracks that God uses to prove whether or not someone or something is really *for you*.' My fiancé revealed to me what was really inside of him."

Don't be in a hurry. Let God show you over a period of time whether or not this guy is a spiritual partner, or if she will really share in your spiritual priorities.

It also takes time for you to determine who is number one in your life, Jesus Christ or your partner.

Trust

"Why, you little wretch. That's the last time I'll ever trust you. You will never pull anything like this again. In fact, just to make sure, I'm removing your bedroom door. Then your mother and I will always know what you are doing."

Marge was a junior in high school. She had let her boy friend into her room through the window in the middle of the night. Her parents came in and caught them.

Her father was so angry, he did remove her bedroom door. She knew she could never regain his trust. She felt she could not stand to live that way, so she ran away from home. She said, "Have you ever tried to live with someone who did not trust anything you said or did?"

Trust is basic to any relationship. Even in business, people want to deal with someone they can trust. You want to be able to trust your friends. In fact, you probably won't keep a friend who has betrayed your trust. How much more you need to trust your beloved.

I believe that total trust begins with your relationship with God.

Would you like to know one way you might lose your partner if you have really given your life to God? Put your partner first, ahead of God. He will not share his glory with anyone. He may move that person right out of your life to regain first place in your life. On the other hand, he may let you pull away from him to go your own way and suffer the loss of deep fellowship with him.

Everyone dreams of having that "perfect relationship" with someone they love, but you will never have it unless you put your relationship with God first.

An anonymous writer said it this way:

> Everyone longs to give themselves completely to someone to have a deep soul relationship with another, to be loved thoroughly and exclusively. But God to a Christian says, "No, not until you are satisfied, fulfilled, and content with being loved by me, with giving yourself totally and unreservedly to me, to having an intensely personal and unique relationship with me alone, discovering that only in me is your satisfaction to be found, will you be capable of the perfect human relationship that I have planned for you. You will never be united with another until you are united with me exclusive of anyone or anything else."

Trust God

Every facet of your life relationships begins with God, but "without faith it is impossible to please him: for he who comes to God must first of all believe that he is" (Heb. 11:6).

"Oh, good night," you say, "I believe that. Certainly I believe there is a God. That's super basic."

Do you know the rest of the verse? "and that he is a rewarder of them that diligently seek him."

Are you in that process? Are you diligently seeking God?

"Oh, Father, I want your will more than I do mine, or at least I am in the process of moving and growing in that direction." There are some beautiful things waiting for you down the road, if this is your honest attitude.

It was after college that I surrendered my dating life to God. I was working at a teenage dude ranch where we had forty horses, an olympic-size swimming pool, and five hundred acres of rolling hills and lush green valleys.

I finally determined to approach dating the way I believed God wanted me to. I resolved I would only date Christian girls who had similar values to mine. I would look for inner qualities of godly character and not just at outward beauty, and one of my major purposes for spending time with a girl would be to set an example of godliness.

After I set these standards for myself and the girls I would date, I didn't have a date for a year. I didn't see any girls whom I thought demonstrated the characteristics I was looking for. For a while I thought, *Thanks a lot, God. You really know how to treat a person who turns over even his dating life to you.*

I had the mistaken idea that if I turned that area of my life over to God, he would bring the perfect girl into my life. I know now that he may do that. But for some people, his will may be that they live without a partner. Singles can have a special awareness of God's promise to supply all their needs (even if he chooses to ignore some of their wants).

In my case, God brought my beautiful wife into my life, and I recognized that he did care about even that part of me. Now, after more than thirty gorgeous years, we are still so much in love we can hardly stand it.

It took time, but I began to learn that I can trust God with every aspect of my life.

Trust your partner

Obviously it is essential to trust God, but you must also build a trusting relationship between yourself and your dating partner. Try to imagine what it would be like to be married to someone you didn't trust.

Mark and Sally had been married thirteen years before they came to see me. When I asked why they had come for counsel, she said, "I can't trust him. He is always secretive about his finances. He spends more time talking to the woman in the office next to his than he does talking to me. He won't even call me when he is going to be late for supper."

"Look who's talking about trust," he retorted. "I put four thousand dollars in the checking account so she could pay all of our overdue bills. She spent every penny of it but didn't even pay the water bill. I can't even trust her to do her housework when I'm not there to watch her. I have no idea what she does all day."

"Listen, Bob," she sobbed, "because of the way he treated me before we were married, I have never really trusted him. He took advantage of me in our physical relationship. He pretended to be such a fine Christian, but he pushed me to do things that we knew were not right to do until we got married."

If trust is so important, why can't some people trust? Why is it so hard for some people to sincerely trust others? Let's consider some reasons.

Losing trust

Poor self-image. If you happen to be one of those people who has had negative "vibes" or negative input from your parents all of your life, you are probably an insecure person. You may think you are not worth two cents. Or, in your effort to feel worthwhile, you may have thought you could achieve self-worth through some great accomplishment, trying to be especially good at something. Perhaps you have thought if you could make the team, then you would be somebody.

If you have gone this route, you've probably discovered that it is empty and left you dissatisfied. One college professor said to Bob Palmer, "I always thought that if I could earn a doctorate, I would have 'arrived.' After I received it, all I could think was, is this all there is?"

Maybe, as you have looked at others and listened to their comments about themselves, you have gotten a negative picture of yourself by comparison. Your view is distorted. It could be compared to walking into a roomful of distorted mirrors, such as those found at an amusement park. This mirror makes you look like you are about two inches wide and nine feet tall; in that mirror you appear to be two and a half feet tall and four feet wide.

If you are using your parents as a "mirror" to reflect back to you your value as a person, you may be in serious trouble. Not all parents are skilled encouragers.

If you have a low opinion of yourself, you will have difficulty trusting others, especially those who say, "I really care about you." You will find it hard to believe they really mean it.

The only way to develop genuine self-worth is by looking at yourself through the eyes of God. You must understand the value he places on your life. He considers you to be so valuable that he designed you to be a unique individual. There is not another person exactly like you in the whole world. If you will give your life back to him, he will do more with it than you can ever imagine. He made you for something special, but unless you give your life to him you'll never discover what it is.

Wrong behavior in your past. Do you suppose a thief trusts anyone? No sir! He thinks that everybody else is stealing, too. The person who has "messed around" physically thinks that everybody else has too. You know how common this saying is: "Everybody's doing it."

Wrong behavior in your past may cause you to distrust others.

Wrong behavior in your partner's past. If there has been wrong behavior in your partner's past, do you realize that it will affect you? Suppose your partner told you about some immoral activities in which he or she had participated before dating you. How would you respond to that?

I am going to make a statement that you will say is inconsistent. And it is, because I believe there are some basic differences between men and women.

Remember in chapter 2 I stated, "A guy thinks with his glands, but a girl thinks with her soul." This means that each of them will respond differently to most things, especially things having to do with sex. Now, if a girl has been up the biological hand grenade ladder with a previous dating partner, I believe she *should not* tell her current boy friend.

Am I saying that a girl should never tell a guy, even if they are getting married? That's a vital question, and my answer is: *An invitation to marriage is the one exception.* When he asks if she will marry him, she should say, "Before I say yes, I need to tell you that there were some activities in my past that I am ashamed of. I'm sorry, but if you will forgive me and you still want me to marry you, then the answer is yes."

However, if a guy has been up the ladder with a previous partner, and if he is now dating seriously, I believe he should tell his girlfriend, not in detail, just in fact. (Never go into detail about past sexual involvement, "for it is shameful even to speak of those things which are done by them in secret" [Eph. 5:12].)

"Good night! You are inconsistent, Bob. Why should the guys admit it, while the women are supposed to have lockjaw?"

Since a guy "thinks with his glands," he is sexually oriented. He is going after that top rung. Whether he will admit it to himself or not, this is the direction he would love to go. When he learns that the woman he is dating has had sexual experience, most guys will be tempted to pursue the same course. He will probably push her to go as far as she has gone before.

What should a girl say if a guy she is dating asks if she is a virgin? If she is not, should she tell him, or should she lie to him so that he won't pressure her to have sex with him?

She should never lie. She could simply say, "I don't think that is a subject to discuss with anyone except the man I plan to marry."

Why, then, should a man tell the woman if he has been up that ladder? So she can be super cautious on their dates. She will need to be very alert to anything that could lead to physical intimacy. She can put on her "spiritual" armor. "Put on the whole armor of God."

I told you it would be inconsistent.

She was a striking girl. Her blond hair was so long she could sit on it. Before she started dating this guy, she had been to bed with a married man. When she and her fiancé came for counseling, she explained, "I thought intimate friends should not keep secrets from each other, so I told him about it."

He sat right there listening, as I asked, "What was his response?"

"Oh, he looked at me and said, 'Hey, I love you and I accept you for what you are. I look upon you as a virgin. I forgive you. It's as if it never happened, as far as I'm concerned.' "I was so astonished, I could hardly believe it," she added.

But do you know what Satan did with that information later? He worked on that man's mind until the guy came out with this: "Hey, if she has been to bed with someone else, maybe she will go to bed with me."

That's exactly what happened, and sex was the death of love. Her love died; she canceled her marriage plans and broke their engagement.

Wrong behavior in your present relationship. Some people have a hard time trusting each other because of wrong behavior in their present relationships. "Oh, so there is some 'hanky panky' going on in this relationship, huh?"

You plant seeds of either trust or distrust during your dating days. I want that statement to reach out and grab you like an NFL tackle.

What are you planting?

Betrayed trust. Have you ever been deceived by someone you trusted? I have counseled hundreds of people who have had that experience. Something snaps or breaks inside you when a trusted friend violates your trust.

A twenty-seven-year-old nurse said, "I don't think I could trust another man as long as I live."

"What happened that developed this kind of distrust in you?" I asked.

She said, "You haven't heard? You mean you don't know why the pastor of our church is no longer the pastor?"

"No, I don't know," I replied. "Why is he no longer the pastor?"

"Because he was involved with eleven different women in our church."

Building trust

Notice the powerful roots on this tree. When I first saw this drawing, I thought the artist had overdone the roots. They looked all "hairy," like the chest of "Max the Brute."

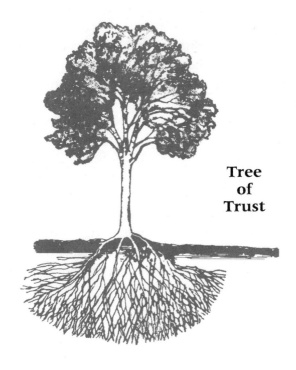

**Tree
of
Trust**

But then I realized that this is the kind of tree that won't blow over in a storm.

Here's how it works. Every time you go out on a date and are faithful to God by applying his principles to your dating relationship, you "water the roots" on "the tree of trust." The roots go deeper and the tree gets stronger.

Your trustworthiness increases in the eyes of that other person. The more she observes you resisting temptation, the more she trusts you. The more you are trusted, the more determined you will be to guard against betraying that trust. That other person's confidence in you becomes stronger, which strengthens your determination to resist enticement. When the strong "winds of temptation" come along and try to blow that tree over, it will probably withstand the test.

There is no iron-clad guarantee that it won't fall. I deal with adultery almost every single day in counseling, and I see that every time you overcome temptation, you are building a stronger resistance to distrust and unfaithfulness.

This is very personal but I, too, have opportunities to add strength and depth to my "tree of trust." I would be less than honest to leave you with the impression I never face temptation.

For my work I do much traveling and am frequently away from home overnight. I meet many people and get into many situations—some ordinary with no tempting overtones, some downright tempting, some unavoidable, some strange. But from my secure knowledge that my wife completely trusts me, I derive great strength for never considering giving in to temptation. When I return home, I tell her everything. She appreciates my openness with her. Our mutual trust is thus renewed and deepened, and our love becomes even more delightful.

12

Becoming Vulnerable

Paul's girl is rich and haughty,
  My girl is poor as clay,
Paul's girl is young and pretty,
  My girl looks like a bale of hay,
Paul's girl is smart and clever,
  My girl is dumb, but good.
Now, would I trade my girl for Paul's?
  You bet your life I would.

What are you looking for in a dating partner? Are you the kind of person who will go out with anyone who is willing to go out with you? Are you like the guy in the poem, always looking at someone else's date and wishing you could trade?

The Enemy and His Weapons

If you don't have some predetermined standards for your dating partners and activities, you are leaving yourself open to attack. You may be vulnerable to some overpowering temptations.

"Man, I'm ashamed of myself," George admitted. "Last

spring I accepted Jesus Christ as my Savior, and then at summer camp I dedicated myself totally to him. I started attending a Christian college this fall to begin preparing for the ministry.

"All the girls in the college seemed to be such fine Christians, I figured I would not have to worry about being tempted sexually. Then I dated Jackie. She practically threw herself at me. She made it very difficult to resist temptation, because she encouraged sex in every way she could. One night on a date, she hurt her leg and asked me to massage it. Before I knew it, things had gone too far.

"I really never expected to be tempted like that at a Christian college. I guess I lowered my guard and left myself wide open to Satan's attack."

George was vulnerable to Satan's attack. He was not prepared to defend himself against the weapon with which he was assaulted.

All of us are vulnerable to such attacks unless we have equipped ourselves with the Christian's full armor. What does it mean to be vulnerable? The dictionary defines it as being capable of, or susceptible to, being wounded or hurt; open to temptation; open to attack.

In this chapter we focus on the problem of being susceptible to temptation. There are certain times when we are more susceptible or vulnerable to sexual temptation than we are at other times. If you are aware of these times, you can be better equipped to resist or avoid them.

Fatigue

Have you ever noticed that when you are tired you more easily get to the point where you really don't "give a rip"? I have a little saying: It's hard to care when you are tired.

If you are working, going to school, and trying to keep up your social life, you may be tired all the time. It's also difficult not to be irritable and touchy when you haven't had enough sleep. For instance, someone says to you, "Good morning!"

You respond with, "What did you mean by that, smart aleck?"

Do you sometimes sit in class or in church and look as though you are agreeing with everything that is being said because your head keeps nodding up and down as you try to fight off sleep? Do you realize this could affect your dating relationship? When you are tired and run down, you begin lowering your guard.

Chemicals

I mentioned earlier that two things that usually go hand-in-hand: drinking or drugs, and sex. When you use chemicals, you are no longer in control of yourself; the alcohol or the drugs are in control.

Ephesians 5:18 says: "And be not drunk with wine, wherein is excess; but be filled with [or controlled by] the [God's] Spirit." The NIV says: "Do not get drunk on wine, which leads to debauchery [depravity, immorality]." God does not want alcohol or drugs to be in control of you. He doesn't even want *you* controlling you. If you invite Jesus Christ into your life, the Holy Spirit moves in with you. God's Spirit actually lives in your body alongside your spirit. He wants to be the teacher, the guide, and the controller.

That's why I believe that every drop of alcohol, or every gram of chemical a Christian ingests, lessens the chance that the Holy Spirit is in control. Then you become more vulnerable or susceptible to attack. Jesus said, "No one can serve two masters. Either he will hate the one and love the other, or he will be devoted to the one and despise the other" (Matt. 6:24 NIV).

Whoever or whatever controls you is your master or boss.

Pressure

Extreme or unusual pressure will cause you to be more vulnerable to temptation.

Have you ever been overloaded with responsibilities, deadlines, expectations, and commitments? You wondered how you could possibly get everything done on time. When you eventually became overwhelmed by the pressure, you felt you just had to have some relief. You wanted to release those pent-up feelings. Or perhaps you completed your work and wanted to reward yourself.

I have known people who have given in to sexual temptation under such conditions. This may not be as common as some of these other circumstances, but it does happen.

Revenge

One woman went to bed with her husband's best friend. Why? To get even with her husband. She took two tranquilizers to get the courage to do it, then walked up to the man and dared him to meet her at a motel. He did.

A teenage friend brought Gini to me for help. She was angry, depressed, and pregnant at sixteen. Her parents were sending her to New York to have an abortion, because it was not legal in her home state at the time.

I said to her, "Did you get pregnant on purpose?"

"Yes," she responded.

"Are you married," I asked.

"I was, but my husband was recently killed in a car accident. This is not his baby I'm carrying," she explained.

"Do you know who the father is?" I questioned.

"Oh, yes. He was my husband's best friend," she answered.

"Why did you get pregnant with this guy's baby?" I inquired.

"I got pregnant for the same reason I got married," she said caustically.

As gently as I could, I said, "Would I be allowed to know why you did that?"

"I'll tell you exactly why I did it. I did it out of revenge," she said stiffly. "It was the best way I could think of to get even with my parents for being so strict."

You see, when you are trying to satisfy your vengeance, trying to "get even" with someone, you can become very, very vulnerable to sexual temptation. In a case like this one, sex becomes a weapon.

Loneliness

Teenage girls love to talk on the phone. It seems they are either waiting for a call or calling someone nearly every free moment. Some girls go through great agony every Friday and Saturday night. They sit and stare at the phone. They may get desperate enough to pray, "Oh, Lord, please let someone call. I don't even care what it looks like, as long as it's a man!" Such girls get tired of sitting home watching TV and having popcorn parties with their parents. They become lonelier and more depressed, either because they are not attractive to the guys or do not know how or care to send the signals that they are available. One twenty-six-year-old woman who came in for counseling had never had one date in her entire life.

On the other hand, have you noticed that some people must always have a partner? They no sooner break up with one person than they immediately take up with another. Saturday night they have a big fight and call off all future activities. Monday morning you see them in school hanging all over somebody else. Why do they do this? Maybe they are just starved for attention and affection.

Did you know that the greatest L problem a girl has is loneliness? She has a major need for companionship. She thrives on relationships.

You already know that a guy's greatest L problem is

lust. But have you caught on that both of these *L* problems can lead to sex? She doesn't want to be lonely. She discovers that she can attract guys by the way she dresses, so she does. She may lower her standards on a date to keep the dates coming, or to encourage that one special guy to keep taking her out. Meanwhile, he has sex on his mind and keeps "climbing the ladder," if not actually then by fantasizing.

Loneliness. The very word carries a crushing weight of gloom for those who have been engulfed by its frequent visits. It causes people to do crazy things (things that seem crazy to us) to overcome its haunting presence. It deprives a person of the strength and courage to go on. It crowds some people to the brink of hopelessness.

It is possible to be alone without being lonely, and it is possible to be lonely even in a crowd. In fact, being in a crowd can make loneliness worse.

If you have experienced this profound darkness of the soul, you understand a little of how Jesus felt on the cross when he cried out, "My God, my God, why have you forsaken me?" (Matt. 27:46 NIV). This was the ultimate loneliness—when his Father turned his back. But God will never do that to you and me, because he did it to Jesus for us, once and forever.

What causes a human being to feel intense loneliness? Where does loneliness come from? People may be lonely because they don't feel loved. There are three primary sources of love. Love comes from God, your family, and your friends.

One thing you can count on is that God loves you. Because he loves you, he will never forsake you. Psalm 27:10 is a beautiful verse: "When my father and my mother forsake me, then the LORD will take care of me."

One guy said, "Bob, I know God is always there for me, but I'm lonely for somebody with skin. I just want a real, live friend."

I believe love always returns to the lover. If you will give love to the people around you, you will be loved in return. If you concentrate on meeting the needs of others, it will drive away most of your loneliness.

Isolation

Isolation makes a major contribution to the problem of vulnerability.

You've probably noticed that when the youth group goes to camp or on a retreat, there are certain couples who always try to get away from the rest of the kids. They constantly endeavor to isolate themselves.

"We've got lots of things we need to talk about," they will explain. "We need some time to be alone because of all these important things we need to discuss."

Most adults who have served as camp counselors and been responsible for a group of kids, have had one turn up missing during a meeting. When the counselor arrives at the camp meeting, he counts to see that all his kids are there and comes up one short.

Oh, oh, better go shake the bushes, he thinks. So off he goes with his flashlight. He looks under all the rocks and behind every tree. Sure enough, he finds a couple out in the darkness away from the camp chapel.

When the two kids see the beam of the flashlight coming toward them, they try to figure out what to say to the counselor. What excuse can they give for being way out here in the dark alone?

Maybe the guy has a real "swift" mind, so he whispers to the girl, "Quick, get down on your knees."

"What?" she asks.

"Hurry, get down on your knees," he urges. And then out loud he says, "Oh, Lord, I thank you for this camp . . . " as the counselor nears.

The poor counselor gets close, hears the guy's voice and thinks, *Aha, there they are.* He swings the beam of his flashlight in the direction of the sound. When he sees that they are "praying," he thinks, *Oh, look at that, they're in prayer. Forgive me for the evil thoughts I had about them.*

I was working at a camp when one of the counselors was missing. The camp director went looking for him. When he found the counselor snuggled up with one of the campers in a car, the counselor explained, "She needed counseling, so we came here to be alone."

Leaders are vulnerable too.

Menstrual cycle

When a girl is ovulating each month, she feels more affectionate and is more prone to respond romantically. A girl needs to be aware of the pattern of her monthly cycle so that she can be prepared to resist her own desires. She may have to fight her feelings particularly if temptation creeps up on her right at that special time of the month.

A negative relationship with father

If a girl has an unhappy or harmful relationship with her father, she will probably be more vulnerable to sexual temptation. Maybe she doesn't even have a father, or at least he is not around. There is a void or emptiness in her life that she longs to have filled by a male. Such a girl may be especially susceptible to relationships with older men.

Brenda had very little respect for her father. She dated guys her own age but felt they were terribly immature. She wanted a guy she could respect.

Art and Brenda were both sixteen and juniors in high school. They had been dating for a couple of years when Art's forty-two-year-old dad started taking Brenda special places. In just a short time, Brenda married Art's father. This is an extreme case, but it illustrates the point.

A conquered heart

A girl can be extremely vulnerable when her heart has been won.

Skip and Becky were students in the university when they came to see me. Becky was concerned about the direction their relationship had taken since they had become engaged. She began to cry as she told about the extent of their sexual involvement. She asked, "Why in the world did I ever give in?"

I knew there were three possible reasons she may have given in, so I explored each of them.

I pointed out that if she had gone up the biological hand grenade ladder with previous dating partners, it would be hard to resist. I explained that many times a girl will go part of the way up the ladder with one guy and then go a little farther with the next one. If she had done this, then it would be easy to move up the ladder when she became engaged.

She looked me right square in the eye, held up her finger, and said, "Bob, until Skip came along, I never let one guy touch me, one time, in one place he shouldn't have."

Now *that* is very unusual in America today. She is some kind of rare woman.

So I asked, "What kind of relationship have you had with your father?"

"I've had a fantastic relationship with my father," she responded. So that wasn't the problem.

What else could be the cause? There was only one possibility left, as far as I could see. Skip had won her heart.

She had enjoyed the dates with those other guys, but no one had ever really captured her heart. Now, for the first time in her life she had feelings for a guy she wanted to express, and she was ready to give herself totally to this one. He wanted to express his feelings to her, so up the ladder they went.

Engagement

Engagement can make a person more vulnerable than almost anything else. You see, the attitude becomes, "I belong to you, and you belong to me. We have exclusive rights to one another. Hey, we are going to get married anyway."

By the way, I don't believe in long engagements—not over six months, because the temptation to get physically involved grows more intense and becomes increasingly difficult to resist.

One woman came in for help because she was wracked with guilt. The cause: premarital sex on the night before the wedding ceremony.

"Do you mean *that* close to the wedding it's wrong?"

Yes. When it's wrong, it's wrong. If you take it out of God's context it will always produce some distressing problems such as guilt, distrust, and a breakdown in communication.

You will have to guard very carefully against physical involvement during your engagement period. A common tendency is to feel that since you are going to be married soon anyway, you might as well go ahead and express your love physically. But the purpose of engagement is to build spiritual intimacy. It is to be a time of getting to know the other person intimately in every other way through sharing dreams, plans, goals, and secrets. It is also the time to plan and prepare for the wedding and to lay the groundwork for your financial future.

I believe some practical ways to avoid becoming physically intimate during engagement would include making a commitment to God and to one another not to go beyond a mutually agreed level of physical intimacy. A couple should also plan not to put themselves into a tempting situation but rather arrange to be with others and not alone. They should avoid being together late into the night. It will help them to be more alert to temptation if they pray together at the beginning and again at the conclusion of each time together. I think each of them also needs to be accountable to another committed Christian of the same sex who will pray for them and with them when temptation is especially strong.

Ignorance about the opposite sex

Do you know much about the opposite sex?

"Yeh, we look different."

Remember the statement I made earlier: A woman thinks with her soul and a man thinks with his glands. A man is more sexually oriented. He tends to be controlled by his drives and appetites. I keep saying this, because I can't emphasize it enough.

Girls, you will have to be alert to this. A guy does not think as you think at all. Consequently, a kiss to him is different, in some (but not all) ways, than it is to you.

Here is one difference.

A couple is out by a crystal-clear lake, with the moon reflecting lazily off the quiet water, while the car radio softly plays romantic music in the background. She is snuggled up in his warm embrace in the midst of a tender, lingering kiss. She's thinking, "Oh, I feel so secure in this hunk's arms. He loves me, I love him, and one of these days we'll be married and have all these cute little rug rats. I'll wipe the snot off their cute little noses . . . "

Meanwhile, he's thinking, "Oooh, does this feel good! More! Press a little harder, baby."

While she is thinking about security and marriage, he's thinking about her body and sex.

If a girl doesn't know this about a guy, then she is going to be very vulnerable, and unwittingly she will encourage his vulnerability. "Oh, he must love me because he is always slobbering on me and trying to nibble on me."

Media Brainwashing

You grab a soda and some chips and park yourself on the floor in front of the TV, and with what you are you bombarded? A "private eye" goes to work for a beautiful client. Seven minutes into the story he is in bed with her, and the sheets are pulled up around their necks. This scene is now very common on network television. Then along comes cable TV, which is even more explicit.

When she came in for counsel, she was eight months pregnant with her second child. She had contracted a sexually transmitted disease from her husband. Consequently, she was grieved over her husband and deeply concerned for her children.

She had recently returned home from shopping and found her husband watching an R-rated movie on cable TV in which a woman was being raped. Their four-year-old child was standing in front of the TV, watching. She begged her husband to turn it off, but he refused.

Research shows that even small children are influenced by the sex on television. The subtle power of innuendoes in entertainment conditions us to accept things that were previously unacceptable. The first time you see something it may shock you, but it will not make as much impact on you the second time. Each time you see it you are less disturbed by it. Eventually you may be oblivious to its presence.

I have stayed in major hotels where you can watch X-rated movies on TV, right in your room. All you have to do is call the desk. They connect your TV into the movie cable and add a charge to your room. (No, I've never watched any.)

There are now videos for sale that actually show couples having sexual relations.

Why have people done this? For money. They know what "gets to" men, so they have used it to make money. Women sell their bodies to photographers and "sexual athletes" just to have money.

One X-rated movie was very popular in the late seventies. It cost twenty-five thousand dollars to make and earned well over fifty million. Twenty-five hundred students turned out to see it when it was shown at a major university in Pennsylvania. What was the purpose in showing it to students? To earn big bucks for its promoters.

"For the love of money is a root of all kinds of evil" (1 Timothy 6:10 NIV).

Spiritual Armor

He was about eleven years old when his father put a gun in his own mouth and pulled the trigger. This caused Kevin to feel rejected and unloved by his father. Once, in his late twenties, he wanted to do something kind for his mother, so he cleaned the kitchen very thoroughly. He could hardly wait for her to see it. He thought she would be very pleased. When she walked in and looked around, all she said was, "I've told you and told you not to leave the dishcloth like that." This made him feel even more rejected and inadequate. Consequently, he found it hard to love others.

When he came to our discipleship meeting, that big six-foot, two-inch guy said, "I've tried and tried to apply these discipleship principles at home, but it sometimes seems impossible. It hurt when my mom said that about the dishcloth, as if she had driven a knife right into my heart. It is as hard to live the Christian life at home as it is at work or school."

One day, this idea hit me: Many Christians have a misconception. In the morning as they prepare to go out into the world for the day, they are thinking, "Now let's see, I need to be ready to face the devil. He will attack me sometime, so I'd better be equipped. I'll apply the principle of Ephesians 6:11: 'Put on the whole armor of God, that you may be able to stand against the wiles [attacks] of the devil.'"

So they put on their spiritual armor and go. Then they come home, take off their armor, and get slaughtered right in their own homes.

"Wait a minute, Bob, I don't need my armor on at home, do I?"

You surely do!

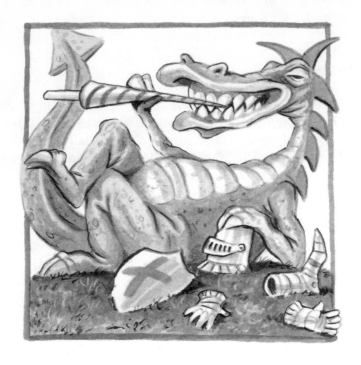

Satan is a master deceiver. He will attack wherever he can. He will use any strategy available to him. He can even give false peace.

One man said, "Bob, my girl friend and I prayed before we had sex, and we had inner peace that we were doing right."

I said, "My friend, you had false peace, which came from Satan. You didn't get that direction from God."

"Now, I don't need my armor on when I am out on a date with a Christian, do I?"

Absolutely!

"Do I need to wear my armor when I'm sitting in church, surrounded by other Christians who believe in the same Jesus Christ I do?"

Oh, yes!

I have been told by many, many people that they have

been wounded by someone in their church. What about you? Have you ever been hurt by someone in your church? Have you ever been tempted by someone in your church?

Both Bob Palmer and I have counseled numerous girls who have gotten sexually involved with a youth leader in their church.

"I don't need my armor on when I am around my family or my best friend, do I?"

I am saying to you that you can't take that armor off, even to go to bed. If you take it off, you will be vulnerable to attack.

Well, what is spiritual armor? Exactly what are we to put on? We are to put on truth, righteousness, peace, faith, and salvation, and carry the word of God.

What God is saying to us is that these qualities are to characterize our lives. If truth and righteousness are to be attributes we possess, or armor we are to wear, how can we give in to immoral activities?

For me to defraud another person, I must deceive. How can I be deceitful if I am wearing truth? How can I be involved in sexual immorality if I am wearing righteousness (God says that illicit sex is unrighteous)?

When you surrender to temptation, you are taking off your armor and handing Satan a victory. I want this to be so obvious to you, to hit you with such impact, that you will never, ever want to take your armor off.

Keep that spiritual armor on constantly. I am praying that you will understand this so fully that it will keep you from ever having sex outside of marriage.

13

I'm So Glad I Waited

A friend of mine was agitated because the flight on which he was scheduled was overbooked. He was forced to wait for the next flight. Waiting was agonizing. He grew more impatient with each digital minute. By the time he boarded the rescheduled flight, his stomach was in a knot; he thought he might be late for his speaking engagement. He wondered why God had allowed him to be bumped from the earlier flight, since he was on his way to preach to several hundred teenagers.

When he arrived at his destination, he learned that the earlier flight had crashed, and all on board were killed. Waiting had saved his life.

Waiting might also save your life. Waiting is never easy. We get instantly impatient in a fast-food line, a traffic jam, or a hundred other daily situations. Patience is not a virtue in the lives of most of us today. Everything about our modern lifestyle encourages instant gratification. For instance, we are persuaded to buy on credit so we won't have to wait for things we want.

I have learned a major lesson in life that has encouraged me to develop patience: *Abstinence is the key to enjoyment*. To abstain means to do without. You don't really appreciate something unless you have been without it.

189

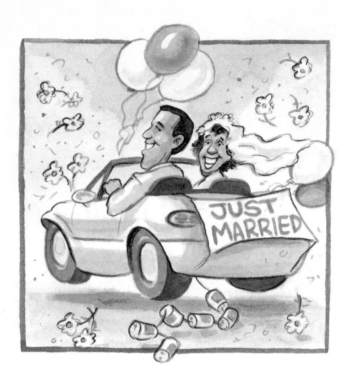

Have you ever been forced to go for a period of time without your favorite food? I once spent eight days in the Canadian wilderness. All we had to eat was freeze-dried food. When I got back to the city, the first thing I wanted was an all-American meal. Hamburgers, fries, and colas had never tasted so good. You don't really enjoy something until you've been without it.

Patience doesn't come easily; it must be developed. And waiting for something is not easy, especially when it is available. All too often sex is available to today's teens, and their natural response is to rush into sex, because they can't see the huge benefits of waiting until marriage.

Because God loves us and wants the best for our lives, we can be sure that his command to limit sex until marriage is for our benefit. The fact that God commanded us to keep sex within the bounds of marriage should be reason enough for us to wait. But just to reinforce this truth in your heart, I have decided to list the potential benefits and contrast them with the possible results of getting involved in premarital sex.

Listed in the left column are benefits you will gain by saving your sexual relationship until after you are married. Listed in the right column are risks you are taking if you give in to sex before marriage. Obviously you would not be hit with all of them, but I can assure you that some of them are universal.

At the same time, there is no ironclad guarantee that if you wait until marriage to express your love sexually you will have a happy, successful union. But the chances of having a lasting, loving, fulfilling relationship are many times greater for those who wait. And if you walk with God and follow his direction, I'm convinced that he will bless you with a beautiful marriage relationship. God made a fantastic promise in 1 Samuel 2:30: "Those who honor me I will honor, and those who despise me shall be lightly esteemed [treated with very little respect]."

Reasons to Wait **The Positive Side**	**Risks in Not Waiting** **The Negative Side**

Personal

Spiritual	*Spiritual*
God commands us to wait	Disobedience to God
Deeper relationship with God	Lose fellowship with God
Potential for spiritual growth	Suffer from spiritual blindness
Pure mind and heart	Increasing sin and its conse-
Major step toward finding God's will for your life	quences
	Impure mind and heart
Clean vessel for God	Accepting God's "second choice"
Proof that God's power and promises work	for your life
	Defiled "temple"
	Spiritual defeat; dishonor God

Mental/Emotional	*Mental/Emotional*
Controlled desires	Controlled and driven by lust
Growing self-control	Lack of self-control

Thoughtful, considerate
High resistance to temptation
Deeply satisfying relationship
Free to respond by choice
Singlemindedness; resistance to other sins
Clear vision to discern real love
Growing self-respect
Clear concept of right and wrong
Enter marriage with a clear conscience free from guilt
Emotional control, gentle, kind, patient
Free of mental, emotional scars: flashbacks, fantasy
Free of grief caused by abortion
Free from resentment
Free from fear of pregnancy, disease, and discovery

Increasing selfishness
Vulnerable to temptation
Unsatisfied, perverted drive
Programmed response
Susceptible to other sins; double-minded
Confuse love and lust
Self-rejection for your past
Foggy sense of right and wrong
Heavy guilt
Emotional instability: angry, explosive, fearful
Chained by emotional, psychological scars
Painful memories, grief
Resentment toward sexual partner
Multiple fears
Deep regrets

Physical
No premarital pregnancy
Free of consequences of abortion
No unwanted child
Body dedicated to God for his glory
Greater potential for more years of sexual relationship in marriage

Physical
Sexually transmitted diseases
Unwanted pregnancy
Consequences of abortion
Unwanted child
Selfish use of "God's temple"
Increased potential for problems of impotence and sterility

Social
No fear of past sin being exposed
Easy to develop deep relationships
Positive reputation
No embarrassment in meeting past dating partners

Social
Stigma of being unwed parent
Constant worry
Afraid to develop deep relationships
Bad reputation
Ashamed to meet past partners

Future
Free to fulfill dreams and plans
Abundant (overflowing) life
Free choices regarding life

Future
Canceled plans, unfulfilled dreams
Limited, disappointing life
Forced marriage, job
School dropout (if pregnancy occurs)

Partner

The joy of sharing a brand-new experience	Nothing new to share
The fun of learning together	Disappointment of past experience
Honesty, no deceit	Deceitful, evasive
Feel appreciated	Feel used
Freedom of growing trust without suspicion	Inability to trust
Growing contentment with mate	Disappointed in mate/marriage
Free to test love on real basis	Love judged on feelings
Transparent relationship	Apprehensive of future relationships
Relaxed relationship	Tense relationship: pressure, demands, anger
Whole self to give to partner	Lost virginity
Pure, joyful wedding	Tainted, forced wedding
Free to marry God's choice	May be forced to marry wrong person
Free from comparison with others	Compare with past partner(s)
Free from jealousy	Jealous of past partner(s)
Increased chance of permanent marriage	Increased chance of divorce
Encourages spiritual intimacy, trust, openness	Lust, discontentment leading to perverted desires
Deepening communication	Blocked spiritual intimacy
Growing desire to meet needs of mate	Shallow relationship
Sex is a delight for both	Little/no communication
Fulfilled spiritually, emotionally, physically	No desire, frigidity, especially in her
Increasing sensitivity to all needs of partner	Sex becomes drudgery
Deep sense of satisfaction	Defrauded, cheated
Builds oneness	Spiraling insensitivity
Proves genuine love	Unsatisfied, insatiable
Gratitude for privilege to express love physically	Prevents oneness
Girl feels free to give self	Love based on sexual feeling
Something special between husband and wife	Resent sex
	Girl feels used, cheap
	Frustration from craving to "go farther"
	Comparison, hurt, insecurity
	Scars: physical, emotional

Child

Born to married parents	Born to single mother
Positive example for child	Child more likely to become unwed parent
Baby's chance of survival higher	
Positive, healthy atmosphere for baby	Chance of infant death
Healthier baby	Tense, negative atmosphere
Loved, unabused child	Unhealthy; low birth weight
Child will do better in school	Resentment; child abuse
Wanted child, reward of love	Problems in school
Natural parent for child	Unwanted child
	Poverty-level existence for most unwed teen moms
	Possible stepparent for child
	Fear of opening up to others
	Loneliness from rejection

Others

Free to love others
Many friends
Free of vengeance
Not responsible for causing others to fall
Giving, loving, unselfish
Happy, open, self-confident
Demonstration of godliness
Parents proud of you
Respect others of like mind
Honorable reputation, respected
Free from shame

What a fantastic list of reasons to wait until marriage for sex. If we live our lives the way God wants us to, we will receive God's blessing, help, and encouragement. He says marriage is to be a lifelong commitment. If you enter marriage with the attitude that "if it doesn't work out, we can always get a divorce," be assured that it will not work out. And you cannot encounter divorce without experiencing devastating consequences for the rest of your life. As I have attempted to illustrate throughout this book, premarital sex is a major contributor to broken lives and marriages.

The Reason Why

God is the designer and creator of life. He is the one who fashioned you to enjoy pleasure and despise pain, to love peace and retreat from conflict. He gave you your emotions, with the desire to laugh and the ability to cry. He fashioned you to be happy and excited when something is fun, and to feel sad when you are disappointed. He designed your body so that you can feel pleasure when someone touches you or you touch them. He equipped you with the ability to become sexually aroused when you are with someone of the opposite sex whom you care about. He built into you the ability to create life in the form of a baby who has the same characteristics the parents possess.

God designed all of this for two major reasons. First, to reveal his glory. He wants us to recognize his power, love, holiness, and all that he is, as we enjoy his creation. He wants us to love him and worship him, and him only. He told us this very clearly.

Psalm 100:3–5: "Know that the LORD, he is God, it is he who has made us, and not we ourselves; we are his people and the sheep of his pasture. Enter into his gates with thanksgiving, and into his courts with praise. Be thankful to him, and bless his name. For the LORD is good; his mercy is everlasting, and his truth endures to all generations."

Second, he gave us these gifts because he wants us to love life and live it to the fullest. He said that he wants us to have an abundant life. Doesn't it make sense that he gave us pleasure? He created happiness and designed us to search for happiness all of our lives.

"Every good gift and every perfect gift is from above, and comes down from the Father of lights" (James 1:17). It's as one little guy said: "God don't make no junk."

You were created to be special. There is no one else in the world just like you. God gave you a unique combination of abilities, gifts, and talents that are different from anyone else's.

I believe there are some special things you can do in your own distinctive way to make an impact on the world that will otherwise be left undone. There are certain people whose lives you can touch who will be influenced for eternity. The only stipulation is that you give yourself totally to God and do all that you do for his glory.

In all of this, sex seems to be somewhat of a pivotal point, because sex can add either pleasure or pain. Sex can be constructive or destructive. It can be used to bring glory to God through a deep, loving marriage relationship and the birth of children who will be raised to love and serve God, or it can be used to temporarily satisfy selfish desire and result in long-term pain and emotional damage.

Why the Pain?

Okay then, if God created sex to be pleasurable and he designed our bodies to derive pleasure from sexual activities, why is there so much pain, guilt, and heartache associated with sex?

By now you can see the answer to that one as clearly as I can. God designed sex for marriage only. Way back in Genesis 2:24 God said, "Therefore a man shall leave his father and mother and cleave [be joined] to his wife, and they shall become one flesh." It says "cleave [adhere, cling] to his wife," not just any woman.

In 1 Corinthians 6:18, God warns us to "flee sexual immorality. Every sin that a man does is outside the body, but he who commits sexual immorality sins against his own body." But then in chapter 7, verse 2 he says: "Nevertheless, because of sexual immorality, let each man have his own wife, and let each woman have her own husband."

Now, here's the point. There is pleasure without pain and enjoyment without guilt in sexual love when it is expressed in marriage, if it is entered into with a godly attitude.

You can have this spectacular privilege. When you obey the Lord and follow his guidelines, you can kneel with your mate and together thank God for the gift of sexual love and pleasure. You can enjoy one another and grow closer to each other as you grow closer to God.

In this book I have been trying to help you see that when God created sex he created something beautiful. But Satan has taken God's creation and turned it into something destructive and ugly. Satan has been able to use sex to destroy great men and women, to topple governments, to crush nations, and to ruin the lives of millions of teenagers. He doesn't want you to see it in all of its holiness and beauty, because that would cause you to praise God and draw closer to him.

Satan wants you to see sex from a selfish viewpoint, as a way to have pleasure just for the sake of pleasure: "I want it because it makes me feel good. I don't really care how you feel."

She was fourteen years old, and like most teenagers she didn't feel that she was very attractive.

The speaker at camp was a handsome "hunk." As she watched him with his wife that week, it was obvious to her that they were deeply in love.

In one of his talks he mentioned that his wife had never even kissed another man. He said it was very special to him that she had kept herself exclusively for her future husband. It would remain special to him for the rest of their lives.

That teenage girl thought, *I may not be pretty, but if I could keep myself for my future husband, maybe I would be special to him.* (Actually, she was a very attractive young woman.) She did keep herself sexually pure. As a result, she and her husband now have one of the most beautiful marriage relationships I have ever seen.

She said, "It wasn't easy, but it surely was worth the sacrifice. If I had it to do over, I would definitely do the same thing again. I'm so glad I waited. God's way really is the best way."

"I'm glad, too," her husband told me. "In a time when sexually transmitted disease is running rampant like a raging forest fire and it seems that unfaithfulness is more common than faithfulness, I thank God daily that he gave me a wife who is not only disease free (as I am) but who also has not given part of herself away to other men. She's all mine. I have no need to feel jealous or as if I have been cheated out of her deepest love."

Wouldn't you love to be able to give that kind of gift to your marriage partner some day? You could.

Some people are wise enough to learn from the example of others, while some of us must pay a high price in painful experience to learn everything the hard way.

The Bible mentions this in 1 Corinthians 10:6, 8, 11 (NIV), where God talks about the difficulties and responses of the Israelites in the Old Testament:

> Now these things occurred as examples, to keep us from setting our hearts on evil things as they did. We should not commit sexual immorality, as some of them did—and in one day twenty-three thousand of them died. We should not test the Lord, as some of them did—and were killed by snakes. These things happened to them as examples and were written down as warnings for us.

Remember this: Get experience at the cheapest possible price. It's your decision. You can determine in your heart that you will listen to the counsel of God and learn from the experience of others, or you will go your own way and learn the hard way.

The Final Challenge

I am challenging you, right now, to lay this book aside, to get on your knees before the Lord, and to dedicate your life, your body, and your dating partner, or future partners, to God. Make a commitment to him right now that, with his help, you will save yourself for marriage so that you can really enjoy the beauty of love and sex in a godly marriage.

And while you're talking to God, begin praying for your future marriage partner. Ask God to protect that person from premarital sexual involvement. Pray that he or she will dedicate his or her body to God and will decide to wait until marriage. Make a commitment to God that you will save yourself for that person whom God is preparing for you.

But do you know what? You can't even dedicate your life to God unless he is your Father. He is not your Father unless you have put your faith in his Son, Jesus Christ, and have accepted him as your own Savior.

The Bible says this in Galatians 3:26 (NIV): "You are all sons of God through faith in Christ Jesus." So before you make the useless effort to live your life in a godly way all by yourself, get on your knees before God and ask him to forgive you of all your sin and ask Jesus Christ to be your Savior.

Only after you have done this can you dedicate your life, your body, your dating relationships, and your future marriage to God. And having done these things, look at yourself differently. God does.

Once you have asked Jesus Christ to forgive you and to be your Savior, the Bible says you have been cleansed by his blood. Your sin has been completely washed away. You were washed! You're not dirty anymore. You are now clean. Look at yourself as God sees you: clean.

Have you ever been around a mechanic who was working on a greasy, dirty engine and who had dirt and grease all over his uniform? Did you notice that he was not concerned about getting more dirt on his clothes? It didn't matter, because he was already filthy.

Contrast this with a bride in her brand-new, spotless, white wedding gown, or the groom in a white tux. If she gets even a small grease spot on her dress, it is ruined.

Now that you have been forgiven and washed by God, see yourself as that bride or that groom. You are clean and spotless, spiritually and morally. Even the smallest sin will soil your life.

Therefore, having accepted Jesus Christ and having been cleansed by his blood and having committed your life and your body to him, resolve that you will do all you can to keep yourself from becoming tainted again by sin.

Having made all these commitments to God, determine in your heart to be obedient to him in every dating relationship. Put your "armor" on and don't ever take it off again.

I guarantee, it is worth every ounce of effort.

The Dating Dilemma